PTSD and Folk Therapy

Studies in Folklore and Ethnology: Traditions, Practices, and Identities

Series Editor: Simon J. Bronner, University of Wisconsin-Milwaukee and Elo-Hanna Seljamaa, University of Tartu

Studies in Folklore and Ethnology: Traditions, Practices, and Identities features projects that examine cultural traditions around the world and the persons and communities who enact them. Including monographs and edited collections, the series emphasizes studies of living folk practices, artists, and groups toward a broad understanding of the dynamics of tradition and identity in the modern world.

Recent titles in the series:

PTSD and Folk Therapy: Everyday Practices of American Masculinity in the Combat Zone, by John Paul Wallis and Jay Mechling
Tradition, Urban Identity, and the Baltimore "Hon": The Folk in the City, by David J. Puglia
Jewish Bodylore: Feminist and Queer Ethnographies of Folk Practices, by Amy K. Milligan

PTSD and Folk Therapy

Everyday Practices of American Masculinity in the Combat Zone

John Paul Wallis and Jay Mechling

LEXINGTON BOOKS
Lanham • Boulder • New York • London

Published by Lexington Books
An imprint of The Rowman & Littlefield Publishing Group, Inc.
4501 Forbes Boulevard, Suite 200, Lanham, Maryland 20706
www.rowman.com

6 Tinworth Street, London SE11 5AL

British Library Cataloguing in Publication Information Available

Library of Congress Cataloging-in-Publication Data Available

ISBN 9781793603890 (cloth)
ISBN 9781793603906 (electronic)

For my friend Chris, and for all veterans facing their darkest hours
—John Paul Wallis

For Elizabeth
—Jay Mechling

Contents

List of Figures

Preface

We two authors found each other in the fall of 2011, when Dr. Julie Sze, then chair of the American Studies Department at the University of California, Davis, emailed Jay with a request. Jay had retired from UC Davis in July of 2009 at the end of a thirty-eight-year career teaching in the American studies program. Previously, in 2004, Jay was watching PBS *News Hour* and on a particular day saw that program's weekly scroll, in silence, of the photographs of those in the US military who had been killed that week in the wars in Iraq and Afghanistan. Jay had two thoughts as he watched that sad accounting of the human cost of war for a single week. His first thought was that many of the faces of the fallen that week looked young enough to be his students. His second thought was that, absent a draft (as there was during the Vietnam War when he was an undergraduate student), most of his students were unlikely to be paying any attention to these wars. He resolved then to create a new course, "War in American Memory," to remedy the lack of any courses in the UC Davis curriculum even remotely about these wars, and he approached a colleague, Dr. Eric J. Schroeder, to see if they could team-teach such a course as a large, general education lecture course in the fall of 2005. Schroeder had taught special topics courses on the 1960s and on the Vietnam War in American studies, having written his dissertation at UCLA on literary responses to the Vietnam War. Schroeder eagerly agreed to the collaboration and they taught the course to 250 undergraduates that fall. In subsequent years (2005–2009) Jay taught the course to smaller classes of undergraduates in the American studies program and in the integrated studies program, the residential honors program for high-achieving first-year students. During these years Jay immersed himself in the firsthand literature—fiction, memoirs, and reportage—of wars American have fought, beginning with WWI and coming forward to the present wars.

In the meantime, a former American studies student, Shirley Schaufel, who was an older, returning student in the 1970s and who subsequently built a successful career for herself as a museum curator and documentary filmmaker specializing in California Native American cultures, contacted Jay and asked him to come on board a team she was assembling to create a documentary film and complementary educational programs (including a traveling museum exhibition) focused on The Pathway Home, a treatment program for veterans suffering severe symptoms of posttraumatic stress disorder (PTSD) at the Veteran Administration's hospital in Yountville, CA, in the famed and beautiful Napa Valley. Shirley had learned of the program, called The Pathway Home (founded in 2008), and its important work with veterans (Poole 2010).

Shirley was going to apply for grants from the California Council for the Humanities (now CalHumanities) and the National Endowment for the Humanities, and she needed a humanist on the team of filmmakers and others on the project. Jay eagerly agreed to join the team, providing ideas and language from the humanities for descriptions of the project, and that assignment plunged him into the literature on PTSD, starting with psycho-historian Robert Jay Lifton's fine book, *Home from the War* (1973), based on his interviews and conversations with Vietnam veterans.

Dr. Sze's email, therefore, came at an opportune moment. Even in retirement from teaching, Jay was continuing to read war memoirs, novels, and reportage for his work on the Coming Home project. Dr. Sze knew about the course but not the PTSD project. Her request was simple. "Jay," she wrote, "I have a student who is an American Studies major and who is the smartest student and best writer I have seen among the undergraduates. He is a veteran who served in the war in Iraq and he came to Davis as a transfer student funded by the new GI Bill. He wants to write his senior honors thesis in American studies on his experiences as a Marine in Iraq. Could you please work with him on his thesis?"

Of course Jay said yes and he contacted JP (John Paul).

Our conversations while JP worked on his honors thesis throughout the 2011–2012 academic year proved so rich and rewarding that we decided to collaborate further after JP graduated. JP had been accepted to the UC Davis Martin Luther King School of Law, so he and his family (a spouse and two young children) stayed in the area, making it easy for us to meet often to discuss where next to take our collaboration. A color photograph by war photographer, Tim Hetherington, on the back of the dust jacket on Sebastian Junger's book, *War* (2010), shows rough-and-tumble (R&T) playfighting among the Marines at a remote forward operating base (FOB) in the Korengal Valley in Afghanistan. Junger was embedded as a journalist with the unit at Restrepo (the men named the outpost Restrepo to honor a fallen comrade), accompanied by Hetherington, by then a famous war photographer, who later died covering the fighting in Libya. The photographs he took at Resptrepo fill his book, *Infidel* (2010), and he and Junger created a stunning documentary film, *Restrepo* (2010), from the video they shot during those nine months at the outpost.

That color photograph of warriors engaging in R&T playfighting in a very dangerous place triggered in both Jay and JP intense curiosity; for Jay because of his writing about masculinity and play, for JP because he had experienced many examples of R&T playfighting in the Marines and now wanted to fold his scholarly understandings back on those experiences to understand them outside of the taken-for-grated, everyday reality of life with his Marine buddies. That photograph and the questions it raised led us to write and publish our first collaborative article, "Devil Dogs and Dogpiles," which appeared in the journal *Western Folklore* in 2015. That article, reprinted here as chapter 4, looks at R&T playfighting in the combat zone as a folk therapy for stress and trauma.

While we were working on the playfighting article, we wrote the draft of another article in response to a call for essays for a book on folklore and medicine. We wanted to use the second article to explore our notion that folklore in the military and male friendship groups in the combat zone could be and were used by the warriors for short-term solutions to the psychological and physical symptoms of PTSD. That draft article was very long, too long, and we decided that we really had enough ideas and evidence to abandon the essay project and to write a book-length treatment of the uses of vernacular culture as immediate therapy for PTSD. This is that book.

And at the same time, in response to a call for essays from a friend who was editing a book on rivalries and resistance in the US military, we drafted a long article on recruits' and warriors' uses of their bodies as the sites of "micro-resistance" against the "good order and discipline" of the military. Some of the uses of the body for resistance—notably uses of the skin (tattoos), hair, and dress (including folk drag performances)—likely have their own therapeutic value for the warriors, though we have not dedicated separate chapters in the present book to those folk practices.

The sociologist C. Wright Mills long ago wrote that the function of what he called "the sociological imagination" was to "connect private troubles with public issues" (1959). Our own study of American culture—especially the cultures of male friendship groups in society—serves the same function for us and, we hope, for the reader. In chapter 1 we offer some autobiographical context, using our own boyhoods as evidence of the socialization of American boys in two generations. We also reflect on our own consumption of popular culture narratives linking masculinity and redemptive violence.

Working together on our writing has been an enormously rewarding experience, as we moved from the mentor-student relationship to working as peer scholars. We hope that our collaboration brings something new to thinking about masculinity, violence, the folklore of the small group of warriors, and the impact of American mythologies of war.

Acknowledgments

JOHN PAUL WALLIS

My mentor, friend, and coauthor Jay Mechling, who was critical to my personal assimilation back into civilian life. He is an example of how curiosity and conversation are essential to reveal and heal the bonds that hold our nation together.

My wife Julia, who makes sure that no matter where I've gone or when I come back, I find myself at home.

My father Paul, who made sure I was exposed to music and the arts, and provided me an unrivaled education. He set the standard for what it means to be a dad.

The Marines of Charlie Company, 1st Light Armored Reconnaissance Battalion, who served and sacrificed with honor, courage, and commitment. I am so privileged to have served alongside them.

My UC Davis American studies and Law School classmates and professors, who demonstrated an esprit de corps that made it possible for me to thrive as a student.

My Punahou and Starbucks friends who ecouraged me and accepted me, no matter where I roamed.

The clinicians, researchers, and dedicated men and women of the Department of Veterans Affairs, who serve and sacrifice for those who have borne the battle.

JAY MECHLING

I have been teaching and writing for fifty years, so over that time I have accumulated too many intellectual debts to mention them all here. I have learned so much from colleagues and students, but my most important "colleague" is my wife, Elizabeth Walker Mechling. We met as freshmen at Stetson University, got married there as seniors, and went off to graduate school together. Soon we saw that her training as a rhetorical critic and mine in American studies meshed perfectly, so we began writing together, joking that she wrote the verbs and adverbs and I wrote the nouns and adjectives. She continues to be the person I want to talk with first when I am trying to think through some puzzle.

Working with JP Wallis on this project was a true delight. Had he never asked me to work with him on his senior honors thesis in American studies at UC Davis, this book never would have happened. I have a book knowledge and visual knowledge of what it is like to be a warrior, but JP brought to the project his life experiences, for which there is no substitute.

We are enormously grateful to Simon J. Bronner for his unflagging confidence in this project and for his wise and encyclopedic understanding of the dynamics of folklore, an understanding we consulted many times.

Chapter 4, "Rough and Tumble Playfighting," first appeared as "Devil Dogs and Dog Piles" in *Western Folklore* 74 (3/4): 2015, 275–308. It is reprinted here by permission from the editors of *Western Folklore*.

The snapshots illustrating this book are from the private collections of Wallis and Mechling. The Mechling snapshots are vintage "found photographs." Wallis obtained permission from the others pictured in the snapshots from his private collection.

Introduction

American warriors bring home with them mental and emotional wounds in addition to any physical wounds they bear. It was not until the Civil War that doctors began to attach a name "soldier's heart" to the cluster of symptoms we now call posttraumatic stress disorder (PTSD), but therapists and others note that we can find the symptoms deep in history and in the literature by and about war veterans, in Achilles (*The Iliad*) and in classical Greek plays, for example. After WWI the syndrome was called "shell shock," and after WWII and Korea "battle fatigue." PTSD was first named and the symptoms first described in clinical detail as a result of therapeutic work with Vietnam War veterans, and the first Gulf War and the wars in Afghanistan and Iraq raised public awareness about PTSD, including the sometimes long wait veterans endure to get therapeutic help from the Veterans Administration and other medical services. Veterans' dysfunctional "folk solutions" to PTSD when they get home, from mild to severe cases, are well-known to the public through media coverage of some veterans' drug and alcohol abuse, violent behavior, sexual compulsion, and suicide (twenty-two a day at last count)(National Suicide Data Report 2005–2016).

This book argues that warriors living, working, and fighting in the combat zone have discovered on their own the temporary therapeutic benefits of some everyday practices not formally thought of as therapeutic, practices we might call "vernacular" or "folk." Some of these practices are recognizable genres of folklore; others are not usually considered folklore by professional folklorists, though we argue that they should be considered so. We view these vernacular practices as something like psychological first-aid in the combat zone, practices meant to bring temporary relief for the stress of living, working, and fighting in the combat zone.

This is an interdisciplinary American studies book that uses as its evidence war memoirs, war reportage, documentary film, press photographs, and vernacular photography (snapshots) from WWI to the present wars in Iraq and Afghanistan. As an interdisciplinary book, we use ideas and interpretive approaches from several disciplines, including history, folklore, anthropology, sociology, psychology, gender studies, media studies, visual studies, and more. Writing about gender sent us deep into the sciences, especially neuroscience and evolutionary psychology, and writing about PTSD sent us into that same literature.

This is not a history book, though the firsthand testimony about experiences in war is from the near and far past (WWI). The evidence is ethnographic. Wallis brings to this study his own ethnographic observations as a participant in war (Wallis is a Marine Corps veteran with two tours in Iraq, 2005–2009), but we can treat the memoirs, formal war reportage, and photography as further ethnographic evidence with all the advantages of ethnographic reporting ("I was there, so you can believe me") and all the shortcomings of a report from one person's point of view, especially in memoirs, which are the products of memory and all its failures. Our ability to generalize about the war experience lies in noting a pattern across many stories.

As an American studies book, the "topic" here really is American culture. More specifically, though, we engage here in the study of the social construction, maintenance, and (when necessary) repair of the performance of "normative" heterosexual masculinity as it is understood in American culture. The recent policy changes permitting women to fill combat roles previously officially unavailable to them (though women have been in combat unofficially for years) opens up the possibility of comparing male and female warriors with regard to the issues that interest us here. The evidence on female warriors is still scant—there are fewer than a dozen war memoirs by women, for example, and we have not interviewed any female veterans. Thus, our treatment of women and the value of everyday, vernacular customs (folklore) performed by those warriors for their own stress is far more speculative than for the male warriors.

Another change in the military has been the end of the policy of "don't ask, don't tell," so there are now openly gay, lesbian, bisexual, and even transgender people in the US armed services. Of course, there have always been in the US armed forces people whose sexual identity and practices have not fit the heterosexual/homosexual binary; what changed was that the warriors who did not fit that binary no longer had to hide their identities, though some still did and still do. The substantial body of research in gender and sexuality studies over the past fifty years (longer than that if you go back to Freud and Kinsey) acknowledges that human sexual identity not only varies across populations but also can be fluid in the individual's own life. Moreover, the same research sees sexual practices and their meanings as highly contextual. For example, some men who identify themselves as heterosexual can engage in homosexual sexual acts without changing their declared sexual identity (Ward 2015), which happens often in all-male settings like prisons and the military.

This truth about sexual identity complicates generalizations we make in this book about the small group cultures of male warriors. There are still powerful forces in American culture, from the toys parents buy their sons to the popular culture narratives consumed by boys and teens, all working to construct in American boys a normative heterosexual identity. These forces are showing cracks, to be sure. Title IX of the Education Amendments Act of 1972 changed the contour of team sports in the United States, parents themselves raised during second wave feminism tend to raise sons and daughters with less rigid gender boundaries, and other forces have made many adolescents and young adults far more accepting of the gender and sexual identity fluidity researchers find in young people in the early twenty-first century.

In an era of an all-volunteer military, though, male recruits tend to be drawn from ethnic groups and social classes where the ideas about the proper performance of masculinity tend to be more traditional than the ideas found in other groups. The statistics bear out the demographics of the typical male recruit, but the many war memoirs we have read provide clear testimony about the ideas of the typical male recruit regarding the norms of masculinity. The draft in WWII, mixing ethnic groups and social classes, while maintaining substantial racial segregation, created a somewhat diverse male fighting force in which could be found a substantial range of ideas about male identity and male sexuality (James Jones' 1962 novel, *The Thin Red Line*, is a superb example of this). Student deferments and other means of avoiding the draft during the Vietnam War tended to skew the typical male recruits toward ethnic groups and social classes with more traditional attitudes about the proper performance of masculinity. The absence of a draft for creating a fighting force in the wars in Iraq and Afghanistan means that economic forces make the military seem like a viable option to unemployment or underemployment.

To say "typical" here, of course, generalizes across a great many recruits, but it is the unavoidable business of historians and social scientists to generalize. As historian Walter P. Metzger (1963) put it, from one point of view all human beings are the same; from another point of view all human beings are different. The challenge is to fashion generalizations that capture some useful truths about humans without doing too much damage to individual differences. This is the challenge we take on in writing this book about the social construction, maintenance, and repair of masculinity in American male warriors in the combat zone.

Of course, the variety of ideas about the proper performance of masculine identity brought to the recruiter's office by the typical young man provides the raw material for the buzzsaw that is basic training. There is still plenty of evidence that the everyday life of males in basic training (boot camp) and then in the military enforces a "male code" that is old, traditional, and still rather rigid in its ideas about gender and sexual identity. As we say, generalizing about the ways the vernacular practices of the typical male groups in the military is a very complicated matter, and throughout this book we make every attempt to fashion meaningful generalizations while realizing that they do not apply in all situations and for all men. We are limited always by the evidence we have. What does a gay or bisexual soldier think about the game of "gay chicken" (see chapter 4) when the game spontaneously emerges in the playful downtime at the forward operating base? We have no evidence so we have no idea. We try to be careful with our hunches and speculations.

These comments and cautions about the construction and performance of normative masculinity in the US military face even more complications with the increasing presence of women in all the armed forces, including women in combat roles. Women who choose to enlist in the military know from the outset that they are joining a fraternity, that the institution they encounter is a masculine one. The military is still trying to figure out exactly how to integrate women warriors into units deployed in the combat zone, though it is clear that some female warriors are "all in" the platoon-size folk groups.

The few war memoirs we have from female veterans suggest that those women entered the military already comfortable in male friendship groups. In some cases the women have attributed their ease in male groups to growing up with brothers and growing up as a self-described "tomboy." Some explicitly mention team sports as an experience that familiarized them with male cultures. This was an explicit aim of Title IX (1972), giving girls and young women access to the team sports that play such a large part in creating men's cultures in friendship groups. With increasing numbers of women entering traditional male professions and organizations in the 1960s, the proponents of Title IX wagered that giving women access to the team sports world so important in the socialization of young men would help the women "crack the code" of male bonding in the friendship group. It interests us to see some female war veterans make that connection.

Whatever the reason, women who enter the masculine world of the warrior in the combat zone already understand to some extent the "male code." It remains to be seen how much the presence of the women in military units will change the male cultures of those units even a little. This is a matter beyond the scope of this book, but we do try to speculate where and when we can how a particular generalization we make might or might not apply equally to the women.

In short, while we recognize all of the complications of writing about American masculinity and tread that territory with care, we find it useful to examine the culture of the male friendship group among warriors assuming that all of the pressures from socialization, poplar culture narratives, and the traditional masculine culture of the military aim at creating, maintaining, and (if necessary) repairing a normative heterosexual identity.

CULTURE AND VERNACULAR (FOLK) CULTURE

We have declared here that our "topic" in this book is American culture, but it will not suffice to assume that the reader understands the term as do we. Here, then, is a short introduction to culture and, especially, to the idea of vernacular folk culture.

The anthropologist Gregory Bateson, whose "frame analysis" (1972 [1955]) informs much of our analysis in this book, was fond of telling the story about the computer programmer who queried the computer: "Do you compute that you will ever think like a human being?" The computer worked on that briefly and came back with the answer: "That reminds me of a story" (Bateson 1979, 13). So simple—to think like a human being is to think in terms of stories. Put aside all the fancy definitions of "culture" and, instead, think about culture as the universe of stories we humans tell each other and listen to in order to bring order to our lives and to make our lives as meaningful as possible. Stories help us "make sense" of our experiences, and our "common sense" is "common" both in its everydayness and in its being shared. At least we assume everyone has "common sense," though it turns out that even this is cultural (Geertz 1983 [1975], 73–93),

When we study culture, therefore, including American culture and small group cultures in the military, we study communication. We study the "stories" (broadly understood) people share. Any given day we experience stories coming at us through different "channels," as the communications scholars would put it. Many of the stories we consume are in the mass-mediated, popular, commercial culture, from print media to electronic media. We experience other stories as oral, told to us in face-to-face encounters. Some "stories" are material, implied in the objects we use every day. Warriors in the male friendship group, for example, can communicate their relationships without words but with the things they share, like cigarettes or food.

Perhaps the most important thing people communicate in small groups is not information (instrumental communication) but emotions and relationships (expressive communication). A favored definition of folklore is "artistic communication in small groups" (Ben-Amos 1971), but recently Mechling (2019) proposed to revise this definition to read "emotional communication in high-context groups," recognizing that the most important information we share using the vernacular folk forms has to do with our emotions and the relationships between members who share a lot of experience, "high context."

While we pay attention throughout this book to the role of mass-mediated, popular culture in providing narratives about masculinity and violence, from war films and television shows to first-person shooter (FPS) video games, we are interested in these cultural stories (some worthy of being called mythologies) to the extent that the stories provide a canopy of meaning over the everyday communication of warriors in their small groups. We read the memoirs and reportage and view the visual evidence of the lives of warriors precisely for the details of their small group cultures.

Sociologists, social psychologists, anthropologists, communications scholars, and folklorists study the cultures of small groups. We variously refer to the communication in those groups as folklore or vernacular culture, both meaning the everyday communication in the group. We most often use "folklore" and "folk group," so let us see how to define those two elusive terms. Defining the "folk group" for our study is rather easier, so we begin there (see Oring 1986).

THE MILITARY UNIT AS A FOLK GROUP

For our purpose we are looking at military folk groups where the members have at least the ability to engage in everyday, face-to-face social interaction, even if they interact with some people much more than with others. JP's experience was in the Marine Corps, so let us look at the structure of a Marine Regiment, understanding that each branch of the service has slightly different organization patterns and even different names for the organizational units (http://www.marineparents.com/marinecorps/regiment.asp):

- 4 Marines to a fire team (4)
- 3 fire teams to a Squad (12)
- 4 squads to a Platoon (48)
- 3 line Platoons and 1 weapons Platoon to a Company (192)
- 5 Companies to a Battalion (960)
- 5 Battalions to a Regiment (4800)

These numbers make it clear that the largest practical folk group in a Marine regiment is the Platoon, about the size of most fraternities on a college campus. The Marine builds closer bonds in the Fire Team and Squad, certainly, but the Platoon is small enough to constitute a folk group. When the military brass (higher officers, the organization's "management") talk about "unit cohesion," they are usually talking about the Platoon and the smaller units within it.

The military is what Goffman (1961) calls a "total institution," that is, a formal organization that controls or tries to control all aspects of a member's life in the institution, from sleeping to eating to urinating and defecating. A prison is the most dramatic example of a total institution, but the military (especially life in basic training) comes close. In even the most extreme versions of total institutions there are enough "cracks" in the system of surveillance and control for folk groups and folklore to emerge.

It is difficult but not impossible for male friendship groups, folk groups, in the military to coalesce during basic training (boot camp). During basic training the total institution is working hard to resocialize the individual, reproducing the "primary socialization" that occurs in the family (Berger and Luckmann 1967), erasing every vestige of the individual's previous civilian identity toward creating a new identity, "warrior." Basic training accomplishes this erasure of previous individual identity by making the recruits as uniform as possible—giving them the same haircut, requiring them to wear the same new clothing, stripping them of their given names and substituting nicknames, feeding them the same food according to strict schedules, surveilling their urination and defecation, and everything else that parents do to and for infants and young children in their initial socialization. And yet, even in this highly controlled environment aimed at bonding the recruits to the institution, there are enough cracks in the system for men to get to know each other and to create small male friendship groups during basic training. Once deployed, the smaller units (fire teams, squads, and platoons) can become the primary folk groups for the warriors. Young men arrive at basic training with plenty of experience with the workings of the male friendship group.

Recent changes in the US military, by which we mean the increasing presence of women in roles previously unavailable to them, require us to consider the changing nature of the male folk group in the US military. The military remains a masculine institution and most of our examples in this book are of folklore in the male friendship group. At the same time, we test our generalizations here by speculating on women warriors in the very male folk groups.

VERNACULAR CULTURE, FOLKLORE

We have adopted Mechling's (2019) version of the classic definition of folklore, now understanding it as emotional communication in high context groups, where "high context" means that the people in the group have enough shared experience that their communication can be highly coded, or what folklorists and sociolinguists would call restricted rather than elaborated communication. We have also made the point, to which we shall return often, that the most important "information" communicated by folklore in the small group is about the relationships between the members, relationships marked by trust. Just entering a play frame with a friend or in a group, for example, requires trust, in large part because in the play frame messages do not mean what they would mean in the frame of everyday life.

There remain a few more points to make about vernacular folk culture before we begin the body of this book. First, an important function of many folklore genres is that they address psychological and social anxieties. Primary emotions like fear provide the motive for a great many genres of folklore we find in groups of warriors, as is true in many dangerous professions. Folklorists prefer to talk about "folk beliefs" rather than "superstitions," but no matter what we call them warriors have a great many charms, some behavioral (e.g., knocking a magazine against one's helmet before pushing the magazine into the weapon or the "three on a match" belief from WWI) and some material (e.g., lucky charms) to protect them against the dangers of combat. Some of the traditional folk phrases used by warriors address psychological anxieties. It may seem like odd comfort in the face of irrational deaths in combat, but oft-used phrases like "there it is" or gallows humor attempt to take away the power of irrational death.

Folklore also often addresses social anxieties and tensions in the group. One of the advantages of folklore as a resource for communication is that folk genres are not personal, not the invention of an identifiable person in the group. Whereas the direct criticism of another in the group likely would lead to verbal and even physical conflict, jokes, playfighting, and other genres of folklore can help manage interpersonal relations. Collective meals can bring people together, even if the "foodways" feature play with the MREs (Meals Ready to Eat) in the field rather than a family's Thanksgiving feast. Playfighting can be a stylized replacement for real fighting, and so on. In short, folklore can provide "first aid" for interpersonal relationships as well as for trauma.

THE PLAN OF THIS BOOK

Equipped with the concepts and language of folklorists, and as two people trained in interdisciplinary American studies, we begin chapter 1 with the larger American cultural context of the socialization of boys and young men. We recognize that women are playing increasingly active combat roles in the wars in Iraq, Afghanistan, and now Syria, and we know full well that women experience the symptoms of PTSD at rates higher than the men. Nonetheless, our focus in this book is on male warriors, with speculation about the relevance for women warriors of our observations and analysis. JP's field experience was with other men and the overwhelming number of memoirs and novels are written by male veterans.

Chapter 2 recounts what the neuroscientists and therapists know about PTSD and its treatment. As an interdisciplinary project examining therapeutic approaches to treating veterans with mild to severe symptoms of PTSD, we necessarily consulted the literature in neurology and psychotherapy in order to "reverse engineer" what vernacular practices in the combat zone seem to duplicate established professional therapeutic approaches to treating PTSD. In particular, the warrior practices we focus on—animal companions, rough-and-tumble playfighting, video game play, masturbation, and deep play—all replicate the neurological and endocrinological processes found in prolonged exposure therapy (PET). Although there is no single favored therapy for PTSD (pharmacological and psychoanalytic approaches are others), and although it has its critics, PET does have an established track-record. PET and the vernacular practices we find in the combat zone share this key process: a state of arousal (including the limbic system's fight-or-flight or freeze prompts) and then the discovery that the arousal has not led to injury or death.

Chapter 3 begins our inventory of folk traditions as "folk therapy" by looking at the role of nonhuman animals as part of the folk group. As we shall see, the current use of service dogs in the treatment of severe PTSD leads us back to the ways the warriors in the combat zone use dogs as well as other animals in the same way. Chapter 4 examines rough-and-tumble (R&T) playfighting in the combat zone. Chapter 5 describes the video game play by warriors in combat zones and links the experiences playing video games with the physiological and psychological experiences in behavioral therapy.

Chapter 6 looks in an unexpected place for folk therapy for the stress of living, working, and fighting in the combat zone. We know that one symptom of PTSD in returning veterans is compulsive sexual behavior, as the sufferers seek the physiological arousal of sex to mimic the arousal of combat. Sexual outlets in the combat zone pose many problems. Putting aside rape, which is not about sex but about power (and there are rapes of American warriors by other warriors), consensual sexual relations violate military regulations. Some memoirs and other evidence suggests that there are opportunities for consensual sexual relations between two men, two women, and a man and a woman in the combat zone, but those carry great risk. Masturbation appears to be the main sexual outlet for warriors, both male and female. So we have included this chapter on masturbation as a folk custom that has some therapeutic value in the combat zone. We feel confident we are breaking new ground here, and it turns out that thinking about masturbation as a folk practice actually leads to some interesting insights into the ways warriors use their bodies to resist the control exercise by the military as a total institution.

Chapter 7 uses the concepts of dark play (as in gallows humor) and deep play to show the "darker" side of folk traditions in the combat zone. These forms of play, as we shall see, touch the deep, dark reaches of the human psyche at war. In the extreme versions, the warrior enters the "berserk state" and often to atrocities of war. Dark and deep play fall along the continuum toward the berserk state.

Our conclusion speculates on the implications of our ideas about folklore and the short-term treatment of PTSD, implications that suggest some public policy changes in the government and in the military to free warriors to feel free to use their own resources (their folklore) to help them deal with the stress of living, working, and fighting in the combat zone.

We also speculate in our conclusion on what happens to our generalizations about the social construction, maintenance, and repair of masculinity in the military, given that the most recent recruits, members of the iGen (Generation Z, born after 1995—male and female alike—hold views of sexual and gender identity different from the ideas held by their predecessors, from the baby boomers through the 13th generation (Generation X) through the millennial generation. Cultures change.

I

Cultural Contexts, Trauma, and Therapy

ONE

The Socialization of American Boys; or, from Boys to Men, from Play Soldiers to Real Soldiers

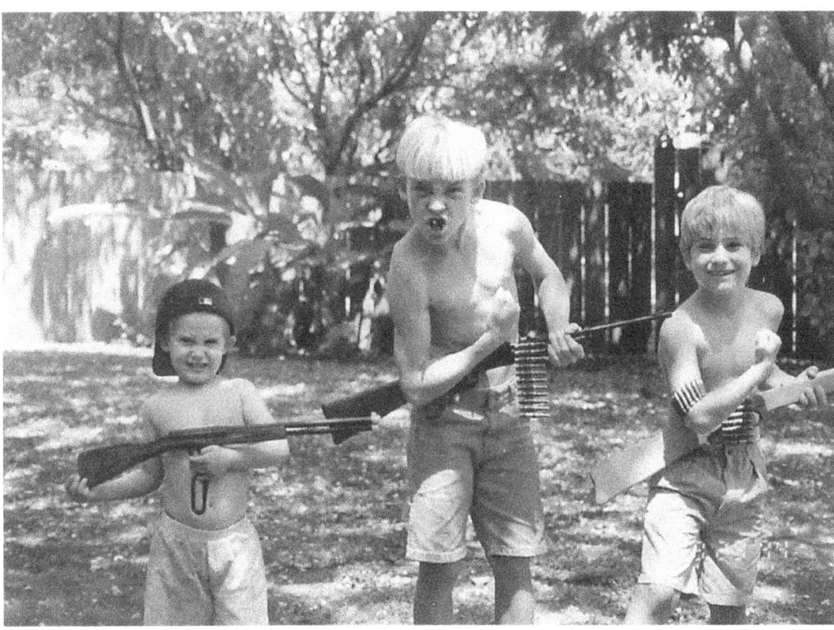

Figure 1.1. Wallis (center), age eleven, with his cousins in Hawaii. Wallis collection.

For us, understanding patterns in the socialization of American boys takes us far in explaining the cultural shape of PTSD symptoms in male US warriors and veterans. Just as patterns in American culture led the United States to fight the Vietnam War the way it did (Baritz 1985) and, doubtless, has led the United States to fight the wars in Iraq and Afghanistan in distinctively "American" ways, so it is that the socialization of American males leads them to understand their individual experiences and their collective experiences in war in terms of shared cultural narratives. These formula narratives about masculinity also help frame the experiences of female warriors and their experiences with PTSD, as we shall see.

We two are American males raised in different generations and want to begin with autobiographical sketches of our own experiences growing up male, especially as those male childhoods absorbed cultural narratives about masculinity and war.

JAY, BABY BOOMER MALE CHILDHOOD

In his memoir about his experiences in the Vietnam War and, later, as an anti-war activist, veteran Ron Kovic (1976) recounts his New York suburban Baby Boomer childhood as an innocent time of his life impelling him toward the war. Like other boys growing up in postwar 1950s white middle-class America, Kovic recalls Saturday afternoon movie matinees where he and his buddies would watch authentic WWII hero Audie Murphy star in his biopic, *To Hell and Back* (1955), and John Wayne in war movies like *The Sands of Iwo Jima* (1949). Kovic and his friends would then go home "and make up movies like the ones we'd just seen or the ones that were on TV night after night" (1976, 65). Sometimes they played war with the countless plastic soldiers bought by the bag full. Sometimes they took their "plastic, battery-operated machine guns, cap pistols" and played in the woods nearby. "We turned the woods into a battlefield," writes Kovic. "We set ambushes, then led gallant attacks, storming over the top, bayonetting and shooting anyone who got in our way. Then we'd walk out of the woods like the heroes we knew we would become when we were men" (1976, 65).

When we were men, becoming heroes. This testimony of a 1950s childhood from this famous, severely wounded Vietnam vet (Oliver Stone made a 1989 film of Kovic's memoir) captures perfectly the socialization of baby boomer boys steeped in the imagined glory of war, and in particular "the Good War." Fast forward decades and we find in the memoirs of veterans of the wars in Iraq and Afghanistan the same testimony about boyhoods filled with playing soldier, imagining the glory of war. Busch (2012), for example, recalls building a play fort in his youth. Daniel Craig (not the actor), a Gulf War veteran interviewed by Messner

(2019, 142) for a book on five veterans working for peace, recalls playing fantasy wars as a kid with "little green army men" and models of tanks and fighting planes and recalls finding "storylines of wartime bravery and heroism" in television shows like *Combat* (ABC, 1962–1967) and films like *A Bridge Too Far* (1977).

Jay was one of those baby boomer children and teens. Born in July of 1945 in Miami Beach, Florida, with only a month of the Pacific War left, he grew up in a 1950s America not unlike Ron Kovic's. Jay was born in Miami Beach because his father was in the army air force. Having married in June of 1940, his parents had moved to Miami Beach from western Pennsylvania in the winter of 1940–1941 for the work (his father was a bartender and waiter). Pearl Harbor the next December 7 and the subsequent declaration of war led the army air force to take over many hotels, public buildings, and even golf courses (as parade grounds) to create a technical training command. Not waiting to be drafted, Jay's father enlisted in the army air force hoping to be a navigator on a bomber. A senior officer, however, discovered that Jay's father had been a bartender in civilian life and decided that the Miami Beach army air force technical training command needed an officer's club in one of the hotels; so Jay's father spent the war tending bar for the army. The practical consequence for Jay was that his father had no war stories to tell, though (to be truthful) a great many of the returning veterans did not talk much or at all about their war experiences in Europe and the Pacific. So many male WWII veterans brought back symptoms of PTSD (then called battle fatigue) and the families of many of those men experienced a husband and father emotionally distant, as described by Friedan (1963) and others writing about middle-class family life in the 1950s.

It mattered little that Jay's father did not regale him with war stories. The mass-mediated popular culture took care of that. Comic books recreated WWII for the millions of boys who read them after the war, and when television entered middle-class homes in the early 1950s (growing from six million sets in homes in 1950s to sixty million in 1960), including Jay's home, the hunger for content meant that cowboy and WWII movies were standard fare on television. The iconic American male, John Wayne, starred in both genres. And it was not just the films. Like Kovic and so many boys in the 1950s, Jay had war toys, ranging from sets of plastic soldiers to toy guns, and (an only child who played alone a great deal) he staged WWII battles with the plastic soldiers, jeeps, tanks, and fighter planes he collected. Images of WWII in popular culture inspired Jay to pretend he was a Marine storming the beaches of Miami Beach. Camping in the wilds of Florida as a Boy Scout provided other jungle scenarios for imagining himself a Marine in the Pacific war.

Jay was an avid reader as a kid and the Landmark Book series, written for boys (one assumes) ages ten to fifteen, provided history lessons to the young readers. Jay recalls reading Richard Tregaskis' *Guadalcanal Diary*

(1955) in the series, and the stories of heroism and tests of manhood under fire fueled his imagination. Boys in the 1950s also had comic books retelling WWII stories, and Jay plunked down his dime at the newsstand near his home for the latest war comic. Put simply, middle-class boys grew up in the 1950s in a culture saturated with images and stories about WWII and, to a far lesser extent, about the Korean War (which had none of the romantic attraction of WWII stories).

On top of the war movies, television shows, comic books, and toys, a whole genre of popular culture texts and toys based on the American West—a heavily mythologized American West—offered boys in the 1950s another stage for the display of rugged masculinity and heroism. Especially vivid in Jay's memory is Disney's 1955 *Davy Crockett, King of the Wild Frontier* theatrical movie, which first appeared in installments (1954–1955) on the Disneyland television show. The last third of the film takes place at the last stand at the Alamo, adding yet another visual narrative about heroism in the face of overwhelming odds in war (see also, Messner 2011).

The Boy Scout experience was a powerful force in Jay's adolescence, and the Boy Scouts provided the structure and male bonding he imagined warriors experienced in the military, especially in war. Student deferments, then a reclassification from II-S (student deferment) to III-A when he got married, and finally a high lottery draft number meant that Jay avoided the draft and never had a military experience. His alma mater, Stetson University in Florida, had an army ROTC unit, and the uniforms and flashy Pershing Rifles drill team tempted him, but he directed his time and energy to other activities. Graduating in 1967, many of his university friends in ROTC received their commissions as second lieutenants and some went off to serve in Vietnam, a war that had heated up considerably by then.

Recently, when having breakfast with a friend his age, the friend asked Jay whether he was sorry he did not do ROTC and experience the military and war. Jay answered, "I think I would have liked it too much." In that answer Jay imagined that he would have loved the army for many of the same reasons he loved the Boy Scouts, and his experience with WWII images and narratives in his childhood planted deep in his mind the notion that combat was the crystalline form of proving your manhood. Knowing that one of the counselors at Boy Scout camp a bit older than he died in Vietnam, Jay knew that there was a great cost to that test of manhood. Yes, he would have liked it too much, and when an anti-war man says that, you know that the power of the "war as a test of manhood" narrative is great.

Even without the test, though, Jay imagined that the military would reproduce the close male bonding he experienced in years of scouting, the bonding that meant he could surrender his own identity to the group and experience the selflessness captured in an unofficial motto used in both the Boy Scouts and military: duty before self. And Jay has read enough memoirs by male warriors to know that it is this feeling of male bonding that is so important and that veterans miss the most, so much that many reenlist to recover that male friendship group they have not found in the return to civilian life.

JOHN PAUL, AN OREGON TRAIL CHILDHOOD

What generation does John Paul (JP) belong to? Scholars of generational birth cohorts have not settled on a single term for the American generation born in the late 1970s and early 1980s. Howe and Strauss (1993, 2000) acknowledge how messy are the borders between generations in their analysis. The millennials, in cohort theory, are the generation born between 1982 and 2000 (hence "millennials"), whereas Generation X (which Howe and Strauss [1993] prefer to call "the 13th generation" for many reasons) was born between the tail end of the baby boomers (1964) and the new baby boom beginning in 1982. But JP (born 1983) and others born in the late 1970s and early 1980s often do not feel they belong to Gen X or to the millennials. Some use "xennial," but increasingly the preferred label is "the Oregon Trail generation," named after the Oregon Trail video games played so often by that birth cohort (Garvey 2015). Howe and Strauss (1993, 14) identify subgroups in the 13th generation according to the popular video game systems they played on—the "Atari-wavers" of the 1960s and the "Nintendo-wavers" of the 1970s—so it seems appropriate to see JP as a member of the "the Oregon Trail generation" (he remembers playing that game).

As a member of the greatest generation, JP's grandfather Vincent joined the army air corps in 1943 as an aviation cadet and was preparing to deploy to the Pacific Theater with his B-25 crew just as another bomber crew dropped "Little Boy" on Hiroshima, instantly killing eighty thousand people and effectively ending the war. The loss of the opportunity to test his mettle in combat showed through in the stories he told about that period. Vincent served through the Korean War and retired in 1964 as a major in the air force. He moved his family to Hawaii, a place they had become familiar with in the years of moving across the Pacific to Korea and Japan. In Hawaii, he worked with the Boy Scouts of America for several years and was eventually offered a position as chief scout executive in Florida. The family was not willing to move, so he turned it down and they stayed on Oahu, where Vince worked as a civil servant at Pearl Harbor, then Hikam Air Force Base.

JP's baby boomer father, Paul, enlisted in the air force in 1971, hoping to take part in the air force bootstrap program to get his degree and become a pilot. Initially stationed in Minot, North Dakota, Paul hated the air force's poor command climate created by career-minded officers.

After two winters in North Dakota, Paul was able to transfer to Hikam, where he would have regular lunches with his dad. Paul deployed to Thailand, where he wrote coordinates for targets for pilots flying bombing missions over North Vietnam. After the fall of Saigon in 1975, Paul was deployed to Wake Island to help with the humanitarian effort assisting Vietnamese refugees, which by his account "was the only time [he] ever saw every single airman, officer and enlisted, pulling on the same rope in the same direction."

Paul began flying lessons while still enlisted, his father helping out when Paul ran out of money, and Paul began working as a commercial pilot even before separating from the air force. In 1979, he was hired by Hawaiian Airlines and built a career in aviation based on his professionalism and flying talent, a point of pride for Vincent. As a single dad, Paul worked hard to provide the best upbringing possible, making sacrifices to send JP to private schools in Hawaii. Sparing his son the rough treatment he had received in public schools in Hawaii as a "haole" (a pejorative term derived from the Hawaiian word for a foreigner, but mostly applied to whites), Paul set a path for his son defined by intellectual curiosity and duty to society.

When Paul was on trips for work, JP stayed with his grandparents, who lived between the two entrances to the Kanoehe Marine Corps Base. Throughout his childhood, JP would go to the marine corps base with his grandfather on various errands, including hunting golf balls on the base course with his cousins. Sometimes the boys would come home with belts of spent brass and links, to be reassembled and worn in bandoliers or hung from their BB guns. JP and his cousins would engage in various battles at their grandparents' house, fielding an arsenal of weapons firing water, corks, rubber bands, BBs, and pellets. There were also medieval swords and shields made from plywood and decorated with duct tape coats of arms. Amazingly, no one was seriously hurt, and no one lost and eye.

Despite the military background, and perhaps in spite of a more martial upbringing of his own, JP's father rejected corporal punishment, emphasized education, and encouraged sports as an outlet for his son. Soccer, baseball, and track were the organized sports of JP's childhood and adolescence. Bodysurfing and boogie boarding were JP's unstructured sports. Athletics were a battlefield growing up, a place of belonging, where potential could be expressed fully. JP excelled in baseball as a middle infielder, but insecurities about failure meant that maintaining a good batting average (where even the best fail most of the time) drove him to quit, a source of great regret.

Soccer was a venue where JP could unleash his body with near reckless abandon. He played with a level of speed and intensity bordering on violence that put opponents on their heels, but that intensity led to repeated injury. In a match against his school's rival, he challenged an opponent for a header in midfield at full speed, bursting the blood vessels in one of the player's eyes. A year later the goalie from the rival school settled the score against JP on a set play in the penalty area. Again challenging for a header at full speed, JP's face was met by the goalie's fist. His face yielded this time, and he was out for the rest of his senior year recovering from reconstructive surgery. JP's identity was challenged, and failing academically he dropped out of high school after his eighteenth birthday.

One of the reasons that sports became a place for the expression of violence was the tension between the lack of violence growing up and violence as a common denominator among American cultural heroes. Action movie stars and Medal of Honor recipients were exalted for their violence. But growing up as a privileged only child, attending mostly private schools, and raised by a father explicitly rejecting corporal punishment, the only appropriate avenue for violence was in sports, which merely reinforced the connection between violence and masculinity (Messner 1992).

Growing up in the 1980s and early 1990s also subjected JP to what Gibson (1994) calls "the New War Culture" in the United States, a culture in which the popular culture narratives were pushing two ideas—that violence in war can be a positive force for justice, and that war is the proper setting for all men to prove their manhood.

After dropping out of high school and moving to California, JP's future was uncertain. Having turned eighteen in March of 2001, September 11th of that year represented a call to arms in the defining war of his generation, the Global War on Terror. At the time he thought being a Navy Seal was the surefire path to honor and manhood, but he was turned down by the navy, having only a GED. The war in Afghanistan would surely be over quickly, just like Desert Shield and Desert Storm, and JP moved on.

When the United States embarked on the invasion of Iraq in March of 2003 to finish the job against Saddam Hussein, JP was determined not to miss out. But living in liberal Marin County, California, he was aware of a strong anti-war sentiment against preemptive invasion of a country on shaky grounds. This was not the acceptably just war against Al Qaeda and the Taliban in Afghanistan, perpetrators and abettors of the September 11th attacks. Despite talking to a recruiter and filling out all the necessary paperwork, friends and family convinced JP to sit out the invasion and he watched the resulting insurgency grow on television.

On JP's twenty-first birthday insurgents hung the burned and mutilated bodies of Blackwater contractors from a bridge, and two resulting battles for Fallujah made it clear that Iraq was a new front in the battle against radical Islam. Al Qaeda may not have been aligned with Saddam Hussein's regime, but the call for Jihad after the US invasion turned Iraq into a melting pot of competing factions of loyalists, terrorists, and tribesmen, supported by various regional powers. It may not have been the war he would have chosen, but there were Americans putting their lives on the line, and violent men who needed to be met with violence. Telling no one, JP enlisted in the Marine Corps in 2005 after having a dream about riding into battle on a horse. He signed a 03XX contract (infantry) and headed for basic training, boot camp.

Many Marine Corps recruits have a point in boot camp where they break down with regret, perhaps in recognition that they have committed themselves to a process and institution that is designed to strip them down and rebuild them with a new identity and philosophy through very deliberate indoctrination. For JP that moment was very positive in that he believed he had been a coward for most of his life, mostly regretting that he had not joined sooner. The Marine Corps provided a new worldview and way of life where violence was not just accepted but encouraged and exalted. In a private conversation with his senior drill instructor (DI), JP was asked why he joined the Corps and, more specifically, why he signed an infantry contract. Recruit Wallis began to give a rote answer embracing the Marine Corps values of "Honor, Courage, and Commitment," but his DI cut him off: "Bullshit! You just want to kill a motherfucker!" Such a motivation would be unsettling in the civilian world, but coming from a DI it was as close to a compliment as a recruit might ever hope to receive.

Following recruit training and the School of Infantry at Camp Pendleton in California, JP received orders for 1st Light Armored Reconnaissance Battalion (LAR). His mentors were Marines who had fought and bled in Fallujah, and they passed on as much knowledge about fighting in urban settings as they could. In March of 2007, JP deployed to Al Anbar Province in Iraq, which had become the Wild West as the insurgency broke out and porous borders allowed for the free flow of weapons, money, foreign fighters, and former Ba'athists of varying loyalty to Saddam, purged from the Iraqi government and military by the United States.

The deployment was largely uneventful but nonetheless transformative for JP and many of his fellow Marines. Unlike the battles fought in cities like Fallujah or Ramadi, 1st LAR would operate mainly in the expansive deserts west of the Sunni triangle, eight-wheel light armored vehicles allowing the battalion to range hundreds of miles throughout the border between Syria and major population centers in Iraq. On one patrol initiated because of some fairly routine intelligence analysis by JP, an improvised explosive device (IED) detonated under the vehicle just behind his. The IED had been initiated with a pressure plate, meaning that several vehicles, including his own, had somehow avoided the IED despite traveling the same narrow path along a washout. Luckily no one was wounded and a second IED failed to detonate.

On a less fortunate day for the Marines in JP's company, Marines in a platoon just a few kilometers away were ambushed while conducting a stop of two suspicious trucks traversing the desert. As the Marines approached, the men in the truck attacked with automatic weapons, rocket propelled grenades, and a suicide bomber. Two Marines were badly wounded, and Lance Corporal Christian Vazquez was mortally injured during the close fight. One of the wounded Marines would earn a Silver Star, the third highest award for heroism in combat for leaving cover to rescue another wounded Marine and suppressing the enemy, despite having been severely wounded by gunfire. Once the Marines on the ground had retreated to the cover of their vehicles, those manning crew-served weapons were able to fire on the enemy fighters, quickly ending the fight with overwhelming firepower.

AMERICAN BOYHOODS, WAR, AND PTSD

Not all of the male American warriors who are the subject of this book played with toy soldiers and toy guns or improvised with sticks as swords and as guns in their physical play at war as boys growing up. Most of the male warriors in the memoirs, fictions, and reportage we rely on here have grown up as boys and then young men in American culture. We make no claim that every boy experiences the same upbringing, but the vast scholarship on American masculinity recognizes patterns in how boys are socialized into men, primarily in the male friendship group. In this chapter we sketch the general outlines of this socialization, in part because the male carries into the military his socialization as a male, and in part because we believe that the socialization of males in American culture frames the therapeutic responses—both folk and professional—to PTSD.

We begin with the nagging question of biological determinism, the central question being how to untangle the role of biology and culture in making American masculinity. We then examine the ways the male friendship group creates, maintains, and repairs as necessary the normative heterosexual male identity the boy is expected to carry into manhood. This journey is far from unilinear, and we attempt to show those complexities and temper the generalizations we want to make, need to make, in understanding the psyche of the male warrior and the dynamics of the folk group in the combat zone.

Male biology and the socialization of boys in male friendship groups are not all that a young man carries with him into basic training (boot camp). As is evident with the movie references made by Kovic and others, and in our own experiences, the mass-mediated popular culture in the everyday lives of Americans creates the narratives (both verbal and visual) that help people make sense of their experiences. As we shall see, television and films and video games and graphic novels provide formulaic narratives for young men to understand what it means to be a man and to understand the relationship between being a man and violent behavior.

We next speculate on how American masculinity aids or hinders the return of the warrior to the "normal" world of civilian life. A constant theme in memoirs and other testimony by veterans is the sudden loss of power and agency in the transition from warrior to civilian. We return to this point in the conclusion.

Finally, we use the existing memoirs by female warriors and some other testimony to examine how the socialization of their male peers affects the female warriors.

THE TROUBLE WITH TESTOSTERONE

Titling this section we appropriated the title of a book by Robert Sapolsky, a primatologist and neuroscientist skilled at explaining to general audiences the dynamic relationship between biology and human behavior, between nature and culture, between nature and nurture (Sapolsky 1997, 2004, 2017). The message from Sapolsky and other evolutionary biologists and behavioral biologists is that the origins of male violence and the particular expression of male violence are complex, not easily reduced to male biology. Still, as Sapolsky says, males "generate an incredibly disproportionate percentage of the violence" in human history (1997, 149), a fact that has received an enormous amount of scholarly and lay attention for many years (Ehrenreich 1997).

There is plenty of evidence that male hormones, especially the category of androgens and anabolic steroids that Sapolsky lumps together (with apologies for simplifying) as "testosterone," made in the testicles, have something to do with male behavior. Testosterone works in the maturing male body to create muscles and secondary sex characteristics, but testosterone also works in the brain and is implicated in male aggression (see also, Courtwright 1996 and LeVay 1993). Lots of clinical and experimental evidence supports the connection between testosterone and aggression. But, and this is Sapolsky's crucial point, "when you examine testosterone levels when males are first placed together in the social group, testosterone levels predict nothing about who is going to be aggressive. The subsequent behavioral differences drive the hormonal changes, rather than the other way around" (1997, 151–52).

Sapolsky looks at his own and others' field research with primates to understand the role of testosterone in the male group, especially the relationship between testosterone levels, hierarchy in the male group, and aggression. The evidence points to the fact that "testosterone isn't *causing* aggression, it's *exaggerating* the aggression that's already there" (1997,

155). So, he concludes: "No biology. No environment. Just the interaction between the two" (1997, 156).

This is the point where the folklorists, historians, anthropologists, and sociologists enter the discussion to try to explain why some societies are very violent and others not. Courtwright's (1996) inquiry into the history of violence in the United States consults evolutionary theory (including endocrinology) and history to argue that young men (ages twelve to twenty-eight) across time and space are the source of most human violence. He rejects simple biological determinism, though. Like Sapolsky, he sees an interaction between nature and nurture (Courtwright 1996, 26).

Our interest in this book is in the American warrior, especially the male warrior, and how the socialization of boys and men in American culture shapes the male friendship group in the military and provides a setting for the warrior's dealing with the stress and trauma of living, working, and fighting in the combat zone.

This initial discussion here of the biology of male aggression will set the stage for our later discussion of the physiology of stress and trauma and our argument about the ways certain folk practices might have a therapeutic effect, at least temporarily ameliorating the symptoms of PTSD.

In the next two sections we explore the American cultural contexts socializing boys and young men into society's norms of heterosexual masculinity. Adolescent boys and young men come to the military with a broad range of sexual orientations and identities, and in our discussions here we must keep in mind the fact that, although the military culture assumes the men are heterosexual, in truth human sexuality is complicated enough that a given man's experience of the military male friendship group will differ according to his sexual orientation, which can also be fluid. In fact, millennials (born 1982–2000) are the most diverse and complicated generation of Americans when it comes to sexual orientation and gender identity (Steinmetz 2017).

The male friendship group is the primary site for the socialization of American boys and young men, so we explore in the next section the workings of such small groups. The boy and young man are also subjected to the larger cultural narratives about masculinity and about violence, narratives to be found in the mass-mediated popular culture of television, film, video games, advertising, and music. To paraphrase Sapolsky—not just biology, not just the boy's socialization in the male friendship group, not just exposure to the larger cultural narratives about masculinity, but the interaction of all of these forces.

GROWING UP IN THE MALE FRIENDSHIP GROUP

The family is the site of the initial socialization of the boy child. The family establishes the "primary socialization" that other institutions—schools, youth groups, sports teams, the workplace, the military, and so on—assume as they undertake the "secondary socialization" of the individual (Berger and Luckmann 1967). The power of primary socialization in the family lies in the emotional environment of the family, for better or worse. This is why psychological and psychiatric therapies usually work so hard at understanding the formative years in the family, where strong emotions cement patterns of behavior and meaning. Many secondary institutions simply assume the foundation of primary socialization and build from there. But other secondary institutions seek to reproduce the emotional power of primary socialization. Fraternities and the military both attempt to socialize the young man by creating conditions similar to the family. That is, they create some version of what Goffman (1961) calls a "total institution," an institution that controls every aspect of the member's body. Goffman's model is the prison or asylum, but the military and fraternities are, too, and a signal that these institutions attempt to recreate the intense emotional bonds of the family in the use of "brother" in both the fraternity and the military (e.g., "band of brothers," as the title of Ambrose's 1992 book has it).

Before they enter these formal institutions, though, most boys have experience in the male friendship group. Whereas girls tend to have a "best friend" and that bond is strong, difficult to repair when damaged, boys' friendship groups tend to be larger and more resilient to damage. Which is to say that boys can have fights one day and be best buddies the next. Boys' friendship groups tend to be hierarchical; boys understand their status and place in the friendship group.

Although male warriors are the primary focus here, this might be the place to anticipate briefly our discussion below about girls' socialization, because over the last thirty years in the United States girls' play has become increasing like boys' play, with all the implications of that for the socialization of girls in their friendship groups. We note here simply that the longstanding pattern of girls' friendships—namely, having a single best friend and looser bonds with other female friends—may be changing.

Among the things boys learn in the friendship group is how to perform stylized aggression. We discussed above the biological basis for male aggression, but we also acknowledged Sapolsky's point that culture shapes male aggression. Parents and other adult caretakers attempt to socialize boys' aggression, but American parents also tend to be tolerant of boys' anger, permitting them that emotion while suppressing others (Stearns and Stearns 1989; Pollack 1998).

Males, especially young males, are capable of intense violence toward others, violence that would destroy the bonds of the male friendship group. Boys learn the usefulness of stylized aggression in the friendship group, "stylized" because it is in the play frame. The value of the play frame is that messages within the play frame do not mean what they would mean in other frames (Bateson 1972 [1955]). Boys acquire the skills of playfighting—both verbal and physical—in the male friendship group. The very existence of a play frame in the friendship group communicates to the participants that they have close relationships of trust. Trading colorful insults, joking, playing practical jokes, pranking, and rough-and-tumble playfighting require the trust of close friends if they are to be "taken" as play. Play frames are fragile, and if they break the participants can repair them if the relationships are important to them. Boys learn all these skills in the friendship group.

Some of these lessons extend beyond the friendship group. For example, playing team sports boys learn that the playing field is one of those framed times and spaces where what happens there does not mean what it means off the field. The play frame of the formal game permits and maybe even rewards stylized aggression, but the stylized animosity on the playing field ends when the players leave the field.

Boys learn in the male friendship what Pollack (1998, 23–25), borrowing from David and Brannon (1976), calls the "boy code." The four injunctions of "boy code" are (1) boys should be "stoic, stable and independent," never showing weakness ("the 'sturdy oak'"); (2) boys are naturally daring, brave, high energy, and violent ("'Give 'em hell'"); (3) boys need to understand their status and seek power and dominance ("the 'big wheel'"); and (4) boys should never express feelings of dependence and empathy, all seen as "feminine" in our culture ("no sissy stuff"). These injunctions stem from the fact that, despite its bravado, masculinity is a fragile social construct and performance, one easily broken and constantly in need of repair.

Masculinity studies turns to feminist psychoanalytic theory to understand the fragility of masculinity, particularly in Western societies. Chodorow's (1978) work is a touchstone for many, as she summarizes so well the theory that mother-raised boys (Mechling 2005) face the difficult developmental task of separating themselves from identification with the mother. Masculinity, therefore, must be defined as "not female," which puts boys and men in the position of having to define themselves as a negative (Frosh 1994). This accounts for the misogyny and homophobia we find so often in the folk cultures of male friendship groups (Mechling 2001, 2005).

As Pollack (1998, 11) and others note, the Boy Code and its constant war against being perceived as feminine is sustained by the cultures of shame and separation in boys' and adolescents' friendship groups. Boys must "prove" their masculinity in the male friendship group. Beneke

(1997) calls the goal of this culture of shame "compulsive masculinity," a masculinity sustained by the tests of "stress and distress," including tests involving physical pain, tests involving psychological pain, and tests by women (1997, 36).

Looking ahead in this book, relevant for understanding PTSD is the Boy Code's admonition that boys should not be allowed to express emotions usually understood as feminine. The one exception, says Pollack, is anger. Boys and girls are socialized very differently in the United States in the expression of anger; simply put, girls are taught to suppress anger while boys are permitted the expression of anger (Pollack 1998, 44). Adults put limits on the physical expression of boys' and teens' anger through violence, of course, but the emotion itself is never considered unnatural and wholly negative in boys; in fact, a certain amount of anger energizes other aspects of the Boy Code, such as competiveness, aggression, and independence (Stearns and Stearns 1986).

Male friendship groups often invent hazing and initiation rituals as a test of manhood and worthiness to belong to the group. Urban, industrialized societies like the United States have lost the elaborate male initiation rituals anthropologists find in other societies (Bettleheim 1954), so boys and young men in the United States tend to "invent" new initiation rituals (Raphael 1988). Male friendship groups like gangs, fraternities, and sports teams find ways to haze, test, and initiate new members, even though in many states and for most formal institutions hazing is forbidden. Many of the invented hazing traditions involve nudity, which in the play frame paradoxically intensifies the male bonding (Mechling 2008c, 2009) because of the trust needed to sustain the frame. In most cases hazing is a test of trust.

Male initiation rituals in the Unites States seem to follow the cross-cultural formula identified long ago by Van Gennep (1961)—stages of separation, liminality (the ambiguous space between two firm cultural categories), and incorporation. The symbolism of death and rebirth is strong in male initiations. The old self separates from the familiar, everyday world to enter a ritual time and space where the old identity dies and the new one is born. The boy becomes the man; the civilian becomes the warrior.

Male initiation rituals in the military have been common for centuries, perhaps the most famous and elaborate being the "Crossing the Line" ceremony (Bronner 2006) on board ships as they cross the equator. Every branch of the military seems to have its own traditions of hazing and initiation, but after some very public and embarrassing events (notably the "Tailhook" scandal of 1991), the military became aggressive in repressing what had become traditional rituals of hazing and initiation. So those rituals went underground.

One element of male hazing rituals we cannot ignore is the strong homorerotic content of the hazing and initiation. Mechling (2008c, 2009) and others detail the homoerotic elements and note the role of these elements in creating strong bonds of trust in the male group. Jane Ward (2015) uses examples from fraternities, the military, and other settings to understand how it is that men who identify themselves as heterosexual have sex with other men and still frame that sex as part of their heterosexual identity. Jane Ward joins Kimmel (2005, 2008) and other scholars writing about masculinity and "sexual fluidity" to observe that even actual homosexual behavior in these settings often actually is in service of another goal—homosocial bonding. Ward makes another point relevant for our focus here, writing that "homosexual encounters between straight white men flourish when adventure and physical endurance is valued over self-image" (2015, 126).

"Physical endurance" is a key phrase in Ward's observation because "tests" imposed by the male friendship group as a step toward incorporation of a neophyte/pledge/"proby" (for probationary member) into the group usually involve physical pain. Enduring pain in the male hazing and initiation is a powerful sign of the masculinity of the neophyte. In basic training (boot camp) a common slogan enunciated by drill instructors is "pain is fear leaving the body," and Wallis (Wallis and Mechling 2015) observes that when he and his Marine veteran friends gather for stories and drinking, the stories always turn to experiences of shared pain and the endurance of that pain.

Ward's focus on actual homosexual acts by men who maintain their heterosexual identities leads her to explain the role of penetration in the initiation rituals, namely, that anal sex "offers men the opportunity to endure homosexual penetration and then stand up, unbroken" (Ward 2015, 164). Mechling's (2008c) analysis of the custom of paddling in male hazing and initiation, though, makes it clear that the *possibility* of penetration in these rituals, not necessarily actual penetration, serves the male bonding goals very well. In some ways the pantomimed anal intercourse we see in male playfighting (e.g., Swofford's 2003 description of the "field fuck"; also Burden 2006, 32) has the same effect of the paddling without penetration—in both cases the bonds are strengthened by the fact that the members *could* penetrate the initiate but choose not to. The penetration is stylized, framed as play, and enduring the pain of the paddling or the pain of the humiliation of receiving the "field fuck" are good-enough tests of masculinity.

So far we have examined the ways biology and the cultures of boys' friendship groups come together to socialize the boy and young man. These small-group experiences, though, also have a larger cultural context, the larger, shared American cultural narratives linking masculinity and violence. The next section looks at those narratives, which really are the mythologies that Americans experience in the mass-mediated popular culture.

AMERICAN CULTURAL NARRATIVES OF MASCULINITY AND VIOLENCE

The socialization of American boys and adolescents into the Boy Code occurs against a larger canvas of cultural narratives about masculinity. Shay (1994, 2002), Tick (2005), Marlantes (2011), and others who see PTSD symptoms as signs of an injury to the soul or character often refer to the mythologies of other cultures in characterizing the models against which American boys and men compare themselves. While most of the relevant mythologies are oral or begin as oral mythologies and end up in print (e.g., Shay's use of Homer's *Iliad* and *Odyssey* as the templates for understanding PTSD in Vietnam veterans), we find America's mythologies in American popular culture, the mass-mediated culture of popular literature, film, television, video games, and music.

As we noted at the outset of this chapter, the baby boomers grew up in the 1950s and 1960s watching WWII films and "playing" WWII in their backyards (Kovic 1976; Wolff 1995). John Wayne was the hero in many of these films, and when the boomers went to war in Vietnam they talked often about soldiers and (more often) officers with the "John Wayne syndrome," which was likely to lead everyone into danger (Lifton 1973, 238). A generation later, Swofford (2003, 64) and his fellow Marines in the first Gulf War consumed both WWII films and Vietnam films, including *The Sands of Iwo Jima* (1949), *Platoon* (1986), *Apocalypse Now* (1979), *The Boys in Company C* (1978), and *Full Metal Jacket* (1987). The American warriors in Iraq and Afghanistan consumed their own set of favorite films, including *We Were Soldiers* (2002), *300* (2006), *Band of Brothers* (2001), *Braveheart* (1995), *Black Hawk Down* (2001), *Enemy at the Gates* (2001), and *Starship Troopers* (1997). Wallis (2012) notes with some irony that "the Iraq war was so long that we were able to watch films about the war we were fighting in," including *Generation Kill* (2008) and *Hurt Locker* (2008).

Even though some of the American war films over the past three decades carry antiwar themes, the young warriors watching these films in the company of other young warriors tend not to see those themes. Instead, they take pleasure in the violence ("the pleasure of the violent films is like the pleasure of cocaine or a good rough fuck," writes Swofford [2003, 64]), in the bonding of the warriors, and in the heroic self-sacrifice within that "band of brothers." The films reinforce the Boy Code internalized at so young an age.

Popular culture narratives tend to be very formulaic. One of the puzzles of mass-mediated popular culture is that people spend money to consume a narrative that is so familiar. The familiarity is comfortable.

Although there are several mythologies we might find in American popular culture, one of the most common American film and television formulae is what Jewett and Lawrence (1977, also Lawrence and Jewett 2002) call "the American Monomyth." We will explain this American

Monomyth shortly, but first we should talk a little mythology and masculinity.

Lawrence and Jewett begin with Campbell's (1949) description of the classic Monomyth in folklore and mythology, the familiar story of the hero quest, wherein the male hero undertakes a journey, encounters and passes several tests along the way, and returns home transformed. This classic formula, which Campbell and other scholars of mythology and literature find in so many cultural traditions, draws its power as a metaphorical account of the maturation of the boy into the man. The formula spotlights "the test" of manhood, which is a feature in many male initiation customs across cultures and which is a feature of the problem of the social construction, maintenance, and repair of manhood or masculinity. Masculinity must be proven by passing tests.

We saw this above in our discussion of the Boy Code and the socialization of boys and young men in their friendship groups. The Monomyth captures perfectly the journey of boys to men, meeting and passing "tests" of their masculinity. Campbell's version of the hero's quest is common enough in the mass-mediated popular culture consumed by American boys and young men. The mythopoetic men's movement of the 1980s and 1990s proposed that a return to the strong male archetypes and mythologies of the past could be the basis for "saving boys" from the weak, feminizing effects of modern life (Mechling and Mechling 1994).

Here is the description of the American Monomyth (Jewett and Lawrence 1977), a pervasive American myth and one that weds religion, masculinity, and violence:

> A community in a harmonious paradise is threatened by evil: normal institutions fail to contend with this threat: a selfless superhero emerges to renounce temptations and carry out the redemptive task: aided by fate, his decisive victory restores the community to its paradisal condition: the superhero then recedes into obscurity. (xx)

In their books Jewett and Lawrence draw on examples from popular culture to demonstrate how pervasive is this American mythology. The film *Shane* (1953) is a perfect example of the formula. One doesn't have to look far to find the formula (e.g., Mechling and Mechling [1999] find it in the 1995 film *Braveheart*). As Jewett and Lawrence describe the American Monomyth, the hero is male, but by the 1990s the female Monomythic hero began appearing in television and film, from Buffy the Vampire Slayer through Ridley (*Alien*) and other female superheroes.

A crucial element for our purposes, and an element that looms in importance when, later, we consider how the mythologies of popular culture negatively affect the warrior's return home and the treatment of PTSD, is the connection the formula makes between masculinity and violence. The "special skill" the American Monomythic hero possesses is violence. Note the phrase "the redemptive task" in the description of the myth. This phrase signals the religious meanings of the violence, an unsurprising element given the ways religion saturates American culture. Slotkin (1973, 1985, 1992) shows how old is the theme of redemptive violence in American narratives, stretching back into colonial stories of Indian captivity to the Westerns of the twentieth century. Slotkin and others rely on Burke's (1973, 106) version of what Burke calls "the representative anecdote" so common in Western literature, the sequence of NEGATIVE - HIERARCHY - GUILT - MORTIFCATION - VICTIMAGE - CATHARSIS - REDEMPTION. Without detailing every stage here, it suffices for our purposes to see that this mythological dramatic structure moves from a paradisal state through the pain of violence to a restoration of the paradisal state, a story of fall (GUILT) and REDEMPTION. The American Mononmyth, then, is a special variant of a mythological structure shared across Western cultures. What shapes the American variant is the deep, long history of violence in American history and the powerful influence of religion—especially Protestant Christianity. Burke's dramatism shows how myth legitimates American violence grounded in religious narratives, seeing violence as a sometimes necessary step toward redemption.

Burke recognizes that the formula he describes is a "secular variant of Christianity" (Rueckert 1982, 133). Bellah's (1967) description of what he calls the American civil religion, a distinctive blend of British liberal political theory and generalized Protestant Christianity, also reflects the role of redemptive violence in American mythologies. Bellah points to Lincoln's second inaugural address in early 1865 as an elegant example of the ways politicians and artists have used the myth to explain episodes of violence in American history. In explaining to the American people why they had to endure the tragic suffering of the Civil War, Lincoln invoked the arc of the representative anecdote. We sinned (human slavery), we suffered, and the necessary violence of the war brings us redemption, returning us to the state of purity we enjoyed before we sinned.

We have taken some time to outline this mythology of redemption and regeneration through violence because American boys and young men are immersed in the formula, which pervades the popular culture they consume, including not just films and television but also video games (Lawrence and Jewett 2002, 199–223). More on video games later, in chapter 5.

As pervasive and influential as the American Monomyth is in defining the masculine hero as a hero suspended in time and space, there emerged in the 1970s a different version of the Monomyth, a version that some critics attribute to the change in the working experiences of middle-class men. Wright's (1977) structural study of American Western films, for example, detects a shift from the singular Monomythic hero—for example, Shane—to the hero as a collection of men, each with a specific talent. The film *The Magnificent Seven* (1960) exemplifies this move to a "corporate" hero in American Westerns after WWII, and that film formula has now persisted for decades, through *Silverado* (1985) and a remake of *The Magnificant Seven* (2016). American young men entering the military from the Vietnam era to the present, therefore, have consumed Western films featuring both solo heroes (the John Waynes, the Audie Murpheys) and collective heroes. We find the same trend in the war films consumed by these American warriors.

We can point to *The Dirty Dozen* (1967) as an early example of the emergence of the corporate hero in war films, though in a sense war films always have featured some version of a "band of brothers." Nonetheless, something did change in the trajectory from *To Hell and Back* (1955) to *The Dirty Dozen* and the films it influenced. Gibson (1994) sees a revival in the 1980s of the idea that redemptive violence can be committed in the service of justice. In this persistent mythology, killing carried the moral meaning of a sacred ritual (Gibson 1994, 102).

Lawrence and Jewett (2002) see the American Monomyth in the video games played by Americans, and although we devote an entire chapter in this book to warriors' play of first-person shooter games in the combat zone, we can pause here briefly to make the point about the pervasiveness of the myth in what the authors call "the latest technomythic platform," the computer (199). In truth, most boys and young men spend far more time playing computer games than they do watching television or going to theatrical films, so if our goal is to chart the pervasiveness of the American Monomyth as a formula narrative linking masculinity and violence with religious legitimacy, then video games are a likely place to look.

What video games offer the player, of course, is the "intense personal involvement in a monomythic scenario" (Lawrence and Jewett 2002, 200), an experience not available watching television or films. The interactive game experience "now allows the participant to *be* a savior and to feel viscerally the pleasures of redeeming a situation from threat" (200). In some games, the player(s) can customize the game "in the direction of personal taste" (200). And there have been even more advances in game design and the technology since Lawrence and Jewett wrote their book.

Lawrence and Jewett posit what they call "the Werther Effect" (2002, 9–10), referring to the widespread, passionate fan phenomenon in response to Goethe's 1774 novel, *The Sorrows of Young Werther*. "In the Werther effect," they write,

> an audience member (a) experiences a work of fantasy within a secular context that (b) helps to shape the reader/viewer's sense of what is real and desirable, in such a way that (c) the reader/viewer takes actions consistent with the vision inspired by the interaction between his own fantasy and that popular entertainment (2002, 10).

If young boys and young men (and girls and young women, for that matter) consume through many media the formula narrative of the American Monomyth, then they might use these experiences as templates for their behavior in other situations, such as combat. Lawrence and Jewett know well the fierce debate among experts and lay adults over the influence of violent media upon children, but they don't feel obliged to settle on one answer or another in the debate over the causes of violence. Instead, they opt for a version of Sapolsky's argument—namely, that video games do not make boys behave violently, but the games do provide narrative structures for the boys' understanding of the legitimacy of redemptive violence. This position suits perfectly our view of what happens when warriors play video games.

We discuss at greater length in chapter 5 the video games American warriors play in the combat zones, a changing menu of games as the wars in Iraq and Afghanistan have dragged on, and the actual ways the warriors tend to play those games as part of their managing social and psychological relationships within the military friendship group. The connection we wish to make here, though, is the presence of the American Monomyth in these fantasy game worlds. Lawrence and Jewett point to the 1980 video game, *Missile Command* (Atari), as one of the first games featuring a "savior premise" (207–9), in this case defending "six cities on the colony planet Zardon from nuclear attack" (207). The plot of this and dozens of other video games in the 1980s and 1990s strongly resembles the American Monomyth. "The endangered-world scenario," they write, "with the innocent being politically unable to face down evil, became a dominant theme in the world of game consoles, arcades and home computers," and in all of the games the hero—the first-person point of view the player takes—is a lone individual (209). The very popular game, *Mortal Kombat* (1995, 1997) and the theatrical films spun off from the game, make the hero a collection of fighters, the same phenomenon Wright (1977) detected in Westerns (Lawrence and Jewett 2002, 218). And the films and games feature the secular religious symbolism we find in other versions of the American Monomyth (219).

AMERICAN MASCULINITY AND PTSD

Chapter 2 lays out what we know about PTSD, current therapeutic approaches to treating PTSD, and the case we are making for understanding folklore in the combat zone as a form of folk therapy more immediate than the long-delayed therapy a warrior receives (if at all) upon the return home. Our long discussion of the role of the American Monomyth in the socialization of boys, however, impels us to make here, even briefly, the link between that socialization and PTSD.

Many therapists treating PTSD in veterans see the toll these American mythologies of masculinity, violence, and heroism take on young men. Psychohistorian Robert Jay Lifton understands that his work with the Vietnam vets really is about "psychological change . . . taking place not in childhood or adolescence but in young adulthood," a stage of life and character development as vulnerable to disruption as the earlier stages (Lifton 1973, 20). Finley (2011, 81) observes with some irony that the familiar PTSD symptoms—social withdrawal, a flattening of emotions, a strong commitment to self-reliance and independence from others—overlap considerably with the masculine traits society expects in its men, traits we also see in the American Monomythic hero. The long-term therapeutic goal for many of the therapists who recognize this tangle of masculinity and violence is to help their patients break free from the expectations of traditional masculinity. And some call for revising the way we raise boys, for setting aside the Boy Code in favor of a more complex, one might say androgynous, masculinity. "Our greatest protection against falling into the thrall of the beast," writes Marlantes (2011, 237), the beast within men that seeks transcendence through violence, "is children raised without shame and suppressed rage." As Lifton puts it, we need to dislodge "the individual and collective sense of honor from the warrior ethos" (1973, 376–77). Making a similar point, in the closing pages of his analysis of the warrior mythology as it reemerged in the 1980s and the hold it has on young men (including JP), Gibson argues that "if paramilitary culture is to be abolished, then other areas of social life will have to be reenchanted" (1994, 306). If American boys need magic and enchantment in their initiation into manhood, then the challenge facing the adults (especially adult men) is to fashion rituals that value honor without violence.

Individual veterans experience PTSD, but many of the therapists and others writing about PTSD in our veterans see American cultural patterns at the root of PTSD, especially the way we socialize boys and young men. This socialization has much to do with why young men join the volunteer military, as is clear in their memoirs and other testimony. The search for excitement and adventure in combat promises a relief from the aimless boredom many feel after graduating from high school. Similarly, many young men crave belonging to a proud group that values honor and integrity, qualities of character they may find in short supply in their male friendship groups and in their institutions of work. Many films portray the camaraderie of the platoon, the close male bonds of friendship and trust. In the films—*Black Hawk Down* (2001) remains a favorite among young men deployed to Iraq and Afghanistan—warriors fight not for mom and apple pie, not for country, not for "freedom." They fight for the warrior to the left, and the warrior to the right. Many young men volunteering to serve in the military are looking for that identity ("A Few Good Men," "An Army of One"), for that affirmation of their masculinity, for the feeling of belonging to a proud "band of brothers," for that initiation under fire from boyhood to manhood. If, as several scholars argue, American culture is more of a "fratriarchy" than a "patriarchy," then these brothers are the touchstone for male values.

Some young men will confess that they also volunteer for combat because they seek the feelings of power over life and death. Vietnam vet Karl Marlantes (2011, 82–88) appropriates Jung's phrase, "the shadow," to name the "enemy within," the deep, dark urge to kill. Grossman (2009, also Grossman with Cristensen 2008) notes that the human revulsion to kill other human beings must be overcome in the training of warriors, but he also notes that training can crack that shell and touch the "shadow." Those who go into basic training knowing that they want to kill another person—preferably a dehumanized "gook" or "haji"—will come out with those skills; and even the recruit who does not recognize or want to recognize his "shadow" will also emerge a killer. Daniel Craig, that Gulf War veteran interviewed by Messner, confessed his discovery of this desire:

> Shit, they're paying me to do this! It doesn't get any better than this. We're killing people. I get to participate in killing people and not get in trouble. It was the ultimate getting away with something, like when I'd steal things or when I would be dishonest and get away with it. It's like using. The dopamine. The adrenaline, all that rush. Here's like, what's the ultimate thing people can do is kill other people. That was the sick part of me, that dark side of me that was like, "Fuck! And they are paying us for this!" (Messner 2019, 153)

The power of deciding who lives and who dies is intoxicating.

All of these motives for the male recruit's joining the military in time of war weave together masculinity and violence, which is what makes the American cultural dimensions of PTSD—both its causes and treatments—so relevant to our search for folk therapies in the field. Masculine identity is fragile, always needing to be proved. So the therapists who write about PTSD as an "identity disorder" (e.g., Lifton 1973), as a "soul wound" (Tick 2005, 5), or as a "soul loss" (Tick 2005, 16) are seeing the American cultural dimensions of PTSD. Traditional masculinity, which is reinforced in basic training, may be necessary for the effective warrior, but traditional masculinity also may not prepare the male for the resilience he needs in combat and in the combat zone. Modern warfare, Tick (2005, 58–61) observes, provides a weak rite of passage for young men, devoid as it is of rich symbolism, ritual, and meaning. The sheer absurdity of modern warfare undermines any young man's expectations that combat will bring mature masculine identity, an identity marked by good character and honor.

We have one more point to make before adding the socialization of women to our cultural analysis. The American Monomyth can complicate the male warrior's homecoming and transition back into civilian life. Many memoirs recount the feeling of impotence when coming back into society. In the combat zone, the warrior has enormous power, including god-like power over life and death. The warrior is the American Monomythic hero using his "special" skill—violence—to dispense justice.

Recall, though, that it is the skill of redemptive violence which, in the American Monomythic narrative, keeps the hero from being absorbed into the society he rescues. Shane rides into the sunset; Superman cannot have a "normal" domestic life; Buffy can never have a relationship with Angel. The American Monomythic heroes are destined to be loners, to float outside of society without hope of settling down, getting married, and having a family. The American hero is suspended in time and space (see Lewis [1955] on "the American Adam").

One symptom of severe PTSD might, indeed, be a tendency to react to frustration with violence. And the pervasive popular culture image of the veteran as a ticking time bomb of violence further isolates the veteran. The veteran ends up experiencing the isolation and separation from society the American Monomyth dictates. This is one reason why so many veterans reenlist, seeking not just the camaraderie they miss but to regain the sense of righteous power they enjoyed when serving in combat. The special skills at violence, so dysfunctional and isolating in civilian life, are functional and valued in the combat zone. The American Monomythic hero is "at home" in the violent conflict.

GROWING UP FEMALE

While most of our evidence fleshes out the lives of male warriors and veterans, the ever-growing presence of women in the US military, including combat roles, obliges us to turn our attention to the women in uniform. The presence of women in the US military is not new. Women have a long, distinguished history as nurses, many times exposed to as much danger as the men they were nursing. According to the Vietnam Women's Memorial Foundation (http://www.vietnamwomensmemorial.org/index2.php), some eleven thousand American servicewomen, most nurses, were stationed in Vietnam during the war. Female nurses and American female civilians were wounded and killed in Vietnam. By the Gulf War (1991), more than forthy thousand servicewomen participated in the war, some in combat roles (Holmstedt 2007, xviii). In the wars in Afghanistan (2001–) and Iraq (2003–), women were playing combat roles even before they were officially open to the female warriors. When Holmstedt published her book, *Band of Sisters*, in 2007, more than seventy American female warriors had been killed and more than four hundred wounded in Iraq (Holmstedt 2007, xix); by 2013, the numbers rose to on hundred forty-four killed and more than eight hundred wounded in Afghanistan, Iraq, and Kuwait (Biank 2013, 5). By all accounts, women warriors suffer the symptoms of PTSD at rates greater than the men, in part because of the high rate of sexual assaults by men who are supposed to be their trusted comrades in arms.

Women who volunteer for the military enter a very masculine institution where the "work product" is violence. What can we say about these women, realizing that our generalizations have the same dangers in writing about women as in writing about men.

Let us return to the issue of biology and aggression, where we started, above, with the men. Having laid out the biology of the "fight-or-flight" response to threats and stress in men, Sapolsky (2004) complicates the story with research by psychologist Shelly Taylor. She and other researchers see a male bias in the research on the endocrinology of stress. Taylor argues that the female response to stress more often is "tend and befriend," a response fueled by oxycotin (Sapolsky 2004, 33). Sapolsky acknowledges that there are controversies over the sex differences in bodily and behavioral responses to threat and stress, and that there are further complications. For example, "sometimes the stress-response in males can be about affiliation rather than fight-or-flight," and an expression of that male response can be strong bonding with other males (Sapolsky 2004, 34).

None of this is to say that women do not experience the "fight-or-flight" response to stress and threats. They have the same endocrine systems as the men, including testosterone made in the adrenals (Sapolsky 2004, 129). We have not found any research on the endocrine systems of women warriors to know if they are more like the men than they are like other women. In any case, we take Sapolsky's point that both men and women can have a range of responses to stress, from the classic "fight-or-flight" to "tend and befriend." One lesson from this is that the folk therapeutic, short-term solutions to PTSD might include intense bonding as well as arousal, something to consider when we discuss rough-and-tumble playfighting in chapter 4. Playfighting may approximate the arousal of combat, but it also stimulates the "tend and befriend" response.

As we saw with boys and men, the biology of aggression and other responses to stress and threat is just the foundation on which culture builds, so we turn now to some observations about the socialization of girls and young women, especially with regard to aggression.

Whereas it is fairly straightforward to look at the socialization of boys in their friendship groups, the socialization of girls in relation to masculinity and violence is far more complicated. We need to look at two settings—the girls' friendship group and the "border crossings" of girls as they enter and are socialized in male friendship groups. First let us look at girls' friendship groups.

Folklorists and social scientists who actually study girls in their natural settings have noted changes over time in the folk cultures of girls' groups. Our evidence of these changes get thinner over time because since the 1980s and the moral panic beginning in that decade about "threatened children" (Best 1990), it has become difficult to study children in their natural settings using fieldwork, ethnographic approaches familiar in the social sciences. Still, there are some generalizations we can glean from the studies.

First, the folk cultures of girls' friendship groups have become more like the folk cultures of boys' friendship groups. Whereas girls' friendships tended to be more dyadic—two "best friends"—and strong, boys' friendships tended to be found more often in hierarchical groups and tended to be more resilient to disruptions, largely because of the stylized aggression learned in the male group, as we saw above, girls' friendship now appear to be more dispersed, departing from the "best friend" pattern and displaying friendship in larger groups.

Now girls' friendships tend to resemble those of the boys, with some notable exceptions (and class and ethnicity play a role in the variations of difference). Similarly, the play of girls has tended to become more like the play of boys over the last few decades. The older view was that girls like cooperative, often domestic play, while the boys liked more competitive and rough-and-tumble play. Thanks to ethnographic work by folklorists (e.g., Hughes 1993, 1999; Goodwin 2006; Beresin 2011), we know that girls actually are as competitive as boys, but they learned to exercise their power indirectly and differently in recognition that they were growing up in a patriarchy where some sorts of power were not available to them.

We can trace to the 1970s and the passage of Title IX of the Education Amendments Act of 1972 the social structural changes that pushed women's small group cultures in the direction of men's. Briefly, thanks to the second wave women's movement of the 1960s and 1970s, women were gaining access to institutions (graduate school, medical school, the management circles in business, and so on) previously open only to men and perhaps to a few women. The women entering these settings and professions dominated by men encountered organizational cultures that resembled the informal culture of the male friendship group. Significant in the socialization of those men were the experiences of boys in team sports. Men in the corporate world often thought and spoke in sports metaphors, and it was in team sports that they honed the performance of stylized aggression and an understanding that what happens in the play time and space of the sports frame does not mean what it would mean in other frames, such as the workplace. This was posing problems for women in the bureaucratic settings, and there arose a large body of advice literature for professional women to help them understand the very male culture of those organizations.

Title IX aimed to remedy young women's lack of experience with team sports, and it has proven to be a successful social experiment. The second wave women's movement in the 1960s and 1970s already was helping push girls' play in the direction of boys' play. Ethnographic study of children's play on school playgrounds, for example, shows that girls' play since the 1980s has become more physical, more aggressive. Whereas elementary school children tended to play in self-segregated groups with only some "crossing" the gender lines in the 1980s (Sutton-Smith, Gerstmyer, and Meckley 1988; Thorne 1993), by Beresin's 2011 ethnographic study of a playground found the girls playing a game called, Sui, short for Suicide, a game similar to handball and dodgeball (Beresin 2010, 44–45). She also found that girls were playing football and basketball, games they were not playing when she studied the same playground in 1991 (2010, 121).

Title IX built on these changing experiences in girls' play such that by junior high school young women were able to play team sports and learn the lessons boys had been learning for a century, including skills in stylized aggression. Significantly, several of the women warriors who have published memoirs of their experiences in Iraq and Afghanistan tell of their own experiences as athletes in high school and college, and one memoirist (Solaro 2006, 243–44) explicitly attributes the fitness of women warriors to their athletic experiences. Some women warriors were raised with brothers and consider themselves "tomboys" familiar with the folk cultures of the boys' friendship groups.

As we did with the boys and men, we have sketched here the biological foundations of women's responses to the stress and threat and we have described briefly the evidence that the play experiences of girls and young women are bringing them ever closer to the experiences of boys and men. What remains is the larger cultural question. How are girls and women raised in the United States influenced by the mythologies linking masculinity and violence?

The American Monomyth began its mythological life with male heroes, but just as the women's movement began changing the ways girls played, bringing more aggression and physicality into girls' play, so the larger, commercial, popular, mass-mediated culture has provided narratives of redemptive violence that girls and young women can consume and identify with. Supergirl, Xena, and similar female heroes were the start, but in *Buffy the Vampire Slayer* (1992 film and television series 1997–2003) young women had a fully drawn Monomythic hero. And young women increasingly play first-person shooter games with brothers, male friends, or with female friends.

We don't have testimony from female veterans to know what effect the American Monomyth has on their return to civilian life. Most of the research and commentary relating to female veterans and violence is about domestic violence where the woman is the victim. It is possible that therapists working with female veterans with PTSD are hearing expressions of isolation and of the burden of dysfunctional capacities for violence felt by those veterans.

TWO

Male Vernacular Culture as Therapy in the Combat Zone

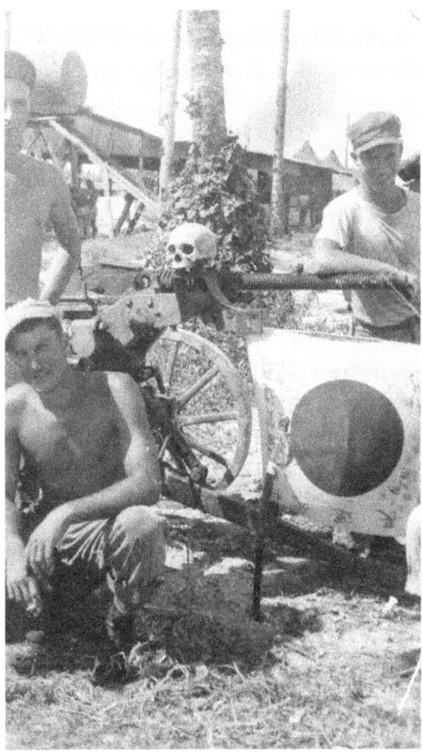

Figure 2.1. Trophies taken from the Pacific, WWII. Mechling collection.

We explore in this book the idea that warriors living, working, and fighting under stressful conditions in the combat zone use their folklore as a form of folk therapy to relieve the stress and even the symptoms of posttraumatic stress disorder (PTSD) that arise in that setting. Just as medics and corpsmen administer first aid to wounded warriors on the battlefield, so the warriors themselves have learned how to use their folklore to provide a kind of first aid for their stress.

This chapter establishes the physiological and psychological mechanisms by which vernacular traditions in the small group of warriors serve therapeutic functions in the short term. The physiological element in the body's and mind's responses to danger and other stressful situations is important for our argument because we believe that some folklore performed in the combat zone by warriors reproduces a common therapeutic approach to PTSD when the veteran seeks professional help upon return home. As we shall see, some folklore performances mimic the physiological arousal experienced in stressful situations, and the short-term therapeutic value of the folk practices lies in the experience of being aroused in a relatively "safe" place and time, without the terrible consequences of arousal in the dangerous time and place of combat.

We begin by examining the uses of folklore as a kind of folk therapy for traumas other than combat trauma. We then lay out the biology of basic responses to stress. Finally, we examine briefly the history of PTSD and of the professional therapies developed over time, beginning in the nineteenth century, and we map the resemblances between the professional therapies and the folk therapies in the combat zone.

FOLK THERAPY

The idea that people use folklore as therapy for stresses in life is not new. Folklorists consider folklore as a resource for living. Everyday life in groups (even alone) is full of both psychological and social anxieties. Folklorists routinely show how folklore addresses these anxieties, even if only for a short while. For example, we allay our fears (a psychological anxiety) with charms and other customs (folklorists tend not to use the term "superstitions"). When tensions arise in our folk groups, we often use stories or humor or customs (e.g., a shared meal) to heal the potentially destructive social tensions. So in our everyday lives we routinely use oral, material, or customary folklore as solutions to "problems in living."

Less routine is the use of folklore as therapy in cases of extraordinary stress, such as the death of a loved one, the dissolution of a marriage, personal illness or injury, and transitions in life (marriage, retirement, dismissal from work, and so on). Folklorists have studied the use of folk arts and crafts as part of the grieving process when a loved one dies. For example, there is a growing tradition of women making "bereavement quilts," a tradition that began within families and then spread to be a commercial folk product, women providing the service of creating a bereavement quilt out of a deceased family member's clothes (MacDowell, Luz, and Donaldson 2018). The most famous bereavement quilt is the AIDS Quilt, a large project begun in 1987 (C. Morris 2011).

Other genres of women's folklore, especially women's folk art and crafts, help individuals and families through difficult times. Folklorists have documented well the uses of family meals ("foodways") to heal stresses and anxieties in families, especially when there are events and forces threatening the cohesion of that group.

Women more often than men are expected to take responsibility for the emotional health of a family or other folk group, especially in times of grief, but men also grieve and some use distinctively male folklore to manage their feelings of loss. Bronner (1996) points to wood carving as a male folk art that some men can turn to when trying to cope with grief or other emotions they are often not free to express.

We count tattoos as a unique form of folk art with therapeutic powers. Although there are amateur, folk tattoos (e.g., in prisons), professionally done tattoos have important qualities as a folk custom, as the customer controls how his or her skin is decorated. Skin becomes a person's "storyboard," as one soldier explains in the 2009 documentary film, *Tattooed Under Fire* (directed by Nancy Schiesari), set in a tattoo parlor near Fort Hood in Killeen, Texas. The film follows male and female soldiers both on their way to Iraq and on their return home. We discuss in chapter 7 the "dark play" (gallows humor) to be found in many tattoos, but here we observe that many of the tattoos shown and discussed in the film memorialized a slain friend. One female soldier featured in a Clark County Historical Museum (Vancouver, Washington) exhibition on "Vet Ink: Military-inspired Tattoos," has "Honor the Fallen" tattooed in an arc at the top of her left bicep, the classic battlefield cross memorial (rifle upside down in boots, helmet on top) tattooed below that, and the initials and death dates of five fallen comrades.

STORIES AS FOLK THERAPY

Storytelling is another folk reaction to stressful events in life, a reaction we can call folk therapy. Famously, Freud and other early psychoanalysts recognized the value of storytelling and invented "the talking cure" as a formal therapeutic method. The folk long ago understood the therapeutic value of sharing stories. In the wake of Hurricane Katrina in 2005, folklorists organized to collect stories from the survivors of that catastrophic storm that flooded New Orleans (Lindahl 2012; Ancelet, Gaudet, and Lindahl, 2013), training some survivors to collect the stories from other survivors, which had positive therapeutic outcomes for both those telling the stories and those collecting them.

Warriors and veterans tell stories, of course. Sometimes they tell stories in the folk group of warriors in the combat zone. Later, veterans gather to share stories recounting their time together. Veterans write war memoirs or short stories or novels. And veterans tell stories in formal therapeutic sessions, either one-on-one with a therapist or in a group. In all its forms, storytelling has therapeutic value for the warrior and veteran. Especially in the combat zone, the warriors' experiences are so random, so irrational, that a story can bring structure and coherence to the chaos and disorder. Stories impose order on troubling experience, even if they are not true.

We do not pay attention here to oral storytelling as a form of folk therapy in the combat zone, in part because this is a huge topic but also because warriors' stories and storytelling has received so much scholarly attention. We focus here, instead, on genres of folklore some readers might not think of as folk therapy for the stress of living, working, and fighting in the combat zone.

We want to make one important point about the power of stories as therapy for stress and its related physical and psychological symptoms before moving on. Folklorists collect and analyze oral performances of stories, which have therapeutic value for both the storyteller and the audience for the story. We need to acknowledge, though, that two other genres of stories can serve therapeutic functions for the warrior—movies and fiction. Although we do not treat these two genres as forms of folk therapy in this book, they are worth a brief discussion.

Thanks to portable media and players, warriors can watch movies in groups or alone when back in the relative safety of the camp or base. We saw in chapter 1 the power of war movies and Westerns as narratives consumed by boys growing up in American culture, and we saw how those movies linking masculinity and redemptive violence provided cultural formulaic narratives for a young man's understanding "what it is like to go to war." Watching movies continues in the lives of young men and women before they enlist and as early as basic training, and a few films turn up often in the war memoirs by veterans of the wars in Iraq and Afghanistan. The film *Blackhawk Down* (2001), based on the 1999 book by Mark Bowden, about the ill-fated military action in Mogadishu, Somalia, commonly appears in accounts of films watched before and after enlisting. David Morris (2015a) writes that in Anbar Province, the Marines there constantly referred to the film *300* (2006), about the Battle of Thermopylae between the Spartans and the Persians, and to *Blackhawk Down*. Wallis notes that the War in Iraq had lasted long enough by the time of his two combat tours there (2007–2009) that he and his fellow Marines could watch theatrical films about the war while they were still fighting it. He remembers watching the HBO seven-part television miniseries, *Generation Kill* (2008), based on the 2004 memoir with that title by Evan Wright.

Stories in print also have therapeutic value. While oral stories clearly count as folklore, we could make an argument that reading novels and short stories, passing around the books, and talking about them with friends serves many of the same functions as does a folk custom. Reading does not reproduce the "flooding" experience of the folk therapies we discuss later in this chapter, but reading can flood the reader awash in emotions, and that has therapeutic value to be sure.

In WWII the Council on Books in Wartime created a special series of armed services editions of books to be distributed free to soldiers serving overseas (Manning 2015). More than 123 million copies of more than 1,300 titles, including fiction and nonfiction, were printed cheaply and in sizes easily tucked into the cargo pockets of uniform pants. American soldiers in the field were reading a broad range of genres, from classics to popular contemporary fiction, from science fiction to mysteries, from poetry to collections of essays.

While we have at least three books (Peisak 2009; Daughtry 2015; Gilman 2016) about the music listening habits of American warriors in Iraq and Afghanistan, there is, as yet, no equivalent study of the books warriors read in those combat zones. The evidence we have from memoirs and documentary films suggests a not-surprising wide range of reading choices. On a blog hosted by AbeBooks, an online used bookseller, active soldier David Abrams (n.d.) provides an insightful narrative about his reading on tour in Iraq in 2005, Abrams reports having his reading interrupted twice by incoming mortar fire, once while reading *Don Quixote* and again while reading Swofford's *Jarhead* (2003). Heller's *Catch-22* (1961) is on Abrams' list (Mechling 1988).

Interestingly, just as Wallis observes that the war lasted long enough that he and his fellow Marines could watch theatrical films about the war while they were still fighting it, Abrams describes reading John Crawford's *The Last True Story I'll Ever Tell* (2005), a novel/memoir based on his experience as a warrior in Iraq. After offering a review of Crawford's novelistic memoir, Abrams reflects on that reading experience:

> It's hard to read about a war while it is still raging on when you lift your eyes from the page. I have no trouble reading about Vietnam (*The Things They Carried*), World War Two (*Catch-22*), World War I (*All Quiet on the Western Front* and *A Farewell to Arms*) or the American Civil War (*The Red Badge of Courage*, which is still on my must-read list), but reading about Operation Iraqi Freedom while the post exchange is still stocking fresh souvenir T-shirts on the shelves. . . well, that makes me anxious and unsettled. (Abrams, n.d.)

Wallis reflects on the novels he and his buddies read in Iraq, Weisbecker's 1986 science fiction novel, *Cosmic Banditos* (reprinted in 2001), was a favorite read and discussed in Wallis's platoon.

Veterans write memoirs, short stories, novels, and even plays. In fact, most of the Greek poets and playwrights were war veterans. Psychiatrist Jonathan Shay reflects on this in his two books—*Achilles in Vietnam* (1994) and *Odysseus in America* (2002)—in which he finds Homer's two classics to be helpful in understanding his therapeutic experiences with Vietnam veterans. The "Theater of War" project, begun in 2009, uses actors to do readers' theater productions of two short Greek war plays for veterans (Healy 2009; Doerries 2015). The plays, both by Sophocles, are *Ajax* and *Philoctetes* and they feature episodes of "the berserk state" in warriors (more on this in chapter 7's discussion of dark play and deep play), which opens up discussion among the readers and veterans after the readings. Shay notes that *The Iliad* has a particularly useful example of the berserk state when Achilles grieves for his slain foster brother (and possible lover), Pátroklos, and enters a "berserk state" resulting in atrocities (Shay 1994, 81–90).

Writing is therapeutic for the veterans, by all accounts, and many veterans often find reading those works by veterans to be therapeutic. Not all do. Some veterans will avoid watching war films and reading war memoirs and fictions, fearful that the experience will rekindle their symptoms of PTSD.

Before closing this discussion of war in theatrical films and fiction, we should mention quickly a popular culture genre that is actually the topic of one of our chapters. Video games have some of the qualities of a theatrical film and create the state of arousal that resembles flooding; hence our treatment of playing video games as a form of folk therapy in chapter 5.

Our discussion here of war "stories" found in theatrical films and in fiction might seem a sidebar to the central discussion of folk therapy for stress and trauma in the combat zone, but we thought it was important to mention these genres of stories beyond the oral because PTSD is primarily an affliction of memory, which includes narrative memory.

Below we survey briefly the current thinking about therapies for treating PTSD in veterans. This is a field beset with controversies, which we are in no position to settle. Most experts in the field of treating PTSD agree that the therapies have to be fashioned to the individual, that not every therapeutic approach works for every veteran.

That said, PET, discussed below, attracts our attention because of all the established therapies used with veterans, this is the therapeutic method that seems to us most like the folk therapeutic strategies we see adopted by the warriors in the combat zone. A fundamental idea driving this book is that warriors do not wait for formal therapy for their PTSD, and formal therapy back home is often delayed for months or even years.

The warriors have discovered a variety of folk therapies, which we describe and analyzes chapter by chapter.

As will be clear in our description of PET, the theory behind that therapy is that the method creates the same physiological responses (fight-or-flight, for example, but even more complex hormonal and brain responses to danger and stress) as do the combat situations that led to the PTSD in the first place. Our hunch, explored in detail in the following chapters, is that folk therapy mimics the more formal processes found in PET, that the folk therapies we examine also create the same physiological and psychological responses associated with the trauma (sudden or prolonged) as does the more formal therapy applied later.

We begin, therefore, with a too-brief discussion of the physiological and psychological responses to the stresses typically encountered in the combat zone. The connections we make between these responses and what we call "folk therapy" is very often speculative, we know. We have some evidence of the physiological and psychological effects of some of these folk therapies—such as playing video games—but we do not have the ideal data on what happens to the brain for each of these folk therapies. Still we believe that the experiential evidence is strong.

One final note. We are mindful of the fact that PET is controversial and does not work as a formal therapy for many veterans, some of whom even report that the therapy worsened their PTSD symptoms. Nonetheless, we believe that the warriors themselves have discovered that the folklore we are calling "folk therapy" give them some relief, however temporary, from the stress of the combat zone. At the same time, we know that some of the folklore is dysfunctional, that some responses to the stress, including drug use and risky play, can be more harmful than helpful in the long run.

THE BIOLOGY OF STRESS

Scientists have studied the physiology of the male body in combat for many years. Neither of us is trained in biology, so we rely here on the work by physiologist and primatologist Robert Sapolsky (1997, 2004, 2017), who writes about the connections between physiology and behavior in ways easily understood by the general audience. We try here to make our discussion of the biology of stress just as readable.

The phrase "fight-or-flight" was coined by Harvard physiologist Walter Bradford Cannon (1871–1945) in his 1915 book, *Bodily Changes in Pain, Hunger, Fear, and Rage: An Account of Recent Researches into the Function of Emotional Excitement*. Other medical scientists have built on this work to give us a full understanding of the chemical and accompanying psychological reactions when a mammal faces a serious threat, such as combat (Sapolsky 2004, 19–36). The sympathetic nervous system in human and nonhuman animals begins secreting various hormones from the adrenal medulla (the core of the adrenal gland), including a family of catecholamines that include norepinephrine and epinephrine (other terms for adrenaline and noradrenaline), which function to "mobilize" the brain and body for action. As Sapolsky (2004, 22) puts it, the sympathetic nervous system "helps mediate vigilance, arousal, activation, and motivation." Other hormones elicited in the "fight-or-flight" (or "freeze," a third possibility) response include estrogen, testosterone, cortisol, dopamine, and serotonin. Sapolsky (2004, 30–32) emphasizes the role of glucocorticoids (steroid hormones) in responses to stress. With the experience of stress or even the anticipation of a stressful situation, a chain reaction moves from hypothalamus to the pituitary gland to the adrenal gland, each gland along the way secreting a hormone that sends to the next gland instructions to secret its chemicals. And important for the parallel with sexual arousal, the pituitary and brain "also secrete a class of endogenous morphine-like substances called *endorphins* and *enkephalins*, which help blunt pain perception among other things" (Sapolsky 2004, 32). Testosterone also plays an important role in the "fight-or-flight" arousal in male warriors who are facing threats. In that aroused state the adrenal medulla produces norepinephrine and epinephrine. The hormones cortisol and neurotransmitters dopamine and serotonin are also involved.

Sapolsky also notes that we don't need to experience a single, dramatic threat for the body's sympathetic "fight-or-flight" cascade of hormonal and neurological events to begin. Even the anticipation, the expectation of a threating situation, can have the same effect. This means that just living and working in the combat zone, even if one is not in immediate danger, can work over time to exhaust the body with "fight-or-flight" physiological responses. Long-term stress actually can change the shape and size of portions of the brain. The amygdala, "the archetypal limbic structure, sitting under the cortex in the temporal lobe" of the brain, is deeply involved in aggression and related emotions and behaviors (Sapolsky 2017, 31). The involvement of the amygdala in aggression, though, can extend beyond the immediate need for a "fight-or-flight" response to danger. Sapolsky notes that "the amygdala expands in size with long-term PTSD" (2017, 34).

A LITTLE HISTORY OF PTSD

The wars in Iraq and Afghanistan since 2001 have meant that as of this writing there are in the United States more than 2.7 million veterans of those wars who have returned home. The estimates are that fully 20 percent of the returning veterans have some level of PTSD. Some returning veterans suffer mild symptoms, while others are nearly incapacitated by the symptoms of severe PTSD. The symptoms of PTSD in general include reexperiencing the traumatic experience, avoidance of stimuli resembling the original traumatic experience, and an exaggerated state of arousal or hypervigilance (McLay 2012, 13).

Some veterans experience PTSD due to a sudden traumatic experience, such as experiencing a life-threatening combat situation or witnessing an extremely disturbing event in combat. Others develop the symptoms of PTSD not through a single trauma but through the prolonged stress of living, working, and fighting in the combat zone. For both, long periods of stress actually change the chemistry and even the architecture of the brain.

The symptoms of PTSD have been familiar in warriors and veterans for a very long time, stretching back into the Greek tragedies and Homer's *The Iliad*. Known as "nostalgia" among Swiss soldiers in the seventeenth century and "soldier's heart" in the American Civil War, the cluster of symptoms now recognized as PTSD was observed as early as the 1860s, when British physician John Eriksen studied "railway spine" in survivors of horrific train accidents (A. Young 1995, 13). The explanation for the symptoms was neurological; hence the emphasis on the spine and nervous system. By the time the well-known psychiatrists—such as Charcot, Janet, and Freud—began treating and writing about the syndrome (Ferenczi et al., 1921), the focus was on memory and the unconscious. These psychiatrists understood the role of diachronic ("across time") memory in constructing a story that made sense of one's own life. The role of therapy, in this view, is to help the patient uncover memories, bring them to consciousness, and diminish their power.

This evolving understanding of trauma met its test in The Great War (WWI). By the end of the war, the Royal Army Medical Corps had treated eighty thousand cases of "shell shock" and other war-related traumas (A. Young 1995, 41). Famed psychiatrist Abram Kardiner worked in a veterans hospital in the United States from 1922 to 1925 and wrote *The Traumatic Neuroses of War* (1941) just on the eve of American involvement in WWII. Where Freud (who wrote very little on war neuroses) saw defensive reactions to wartime trauma, Kardiner saw "adaptive reactions" (A. Young 1995, 89). Traumatic events, explains Kardiner, create such high levels of excitation in the warrior that they disrupt his "ego organization" and he experiences "a sudden loss of effective control over his environment" (A. Young 1995, 89–90). Reaction to the loss of control yields aggression no longer in check by the ego. The new ego which emerges from this turmoil, writes Young in presenting Kardiner's central idea,

> is now thrown into a perpetual struggle to regain mastery and responds in various ways: by adapting itself to a level compatible with its altered resources (making fewer demands on the world, reestablishing infantile relations with the world); by obliterating the problematic portion of the world (introjecting it into the offending body part, which is then paralyzed or anesthetized); or by periodically obliterating the en-

> tire world in order to reestablish amicable relations with it (through syncopal attacks and loss of consciousness, which symbolizes the patient's death and rebirth). (A. Young 1995, 90)

Grinker and Spiegal, in *War Neuroses* (1945), updated the psychiatric thinking about "battle fatigue," as it was called in WWII and in the Korean War (Tick 2005, 99), though their book is mainly descriptive, with an emphasis on "abreactive therapy" for severe cases—a therapy that seeks to have the patient "re-experience the intense emotions which were originally associated with the traumatic battle experiences" (Grinker and Spiegal 1945, 78, quoted in A. Young 1995, 92).

Interest in war trauma waned in the 1950s and it was not until the 1980 edition of the American Psychological Association's *Diagnostic and Statistical Manual of Mental Disorders* (DSM-III), when therapists had gathered considerable experience with Vietnam veterans, that posttraumatic stress disorder entered the official language of symptoms, diagnosis, and therapy. The three necessary elements in the new definition include: (1) the initial traumatic event or events must be unusual, outside everyday experience; (2) observable posttraumatic symptoms, including "persistent and distressful re-experiences of the traumatic event" in dreams, flashbacks, and "intrusive images" and other symptoms now familiar in PTSD patients, including "increased physiological arousal"; and (3) subtypes based on the timing of the onset of symptoms and their duration (A. Young 1995, 107–08; quoted phrases from DSM-III). Jonathan Shay (1994, 2002), the psychiatrist who has worked extensively with Vietnam veterans and has written two books about that work, prefers the label "posttraumatic stress syndrome," avoiding the word "disorder," though he recognizes that we are pretty well stuck with the acronym PTSD.

THERAPIES FOR PTSD

Mental health providers have not settled on a single effective therapy for PTSD. For good reasons, most therapists customize the therapeutic approach to the patient. Below we discuss briefly the most commonly used therapeutic approaches, not because we want to affirm what works best but because we are interested here in the folk therapeutic approaches to combat stress just minutes, hours, and days after the stressful event. Many of the short-term "folk therapy" responses to combat stress resemble the professional therapeutic approaches. Not all folk therapies are effective; some may be harmful. Alcoholism, drug addiction, sexaholism, and risk-taking back home are dysfunctional "solutions" to the anxiety and pain of PTSD (Shay 2002, 39).

At present, therapists treat patients with PTSD with pharmacology (drugs), psychotherapy, or a combination of the two (A. Young 1995, 177). The psychotherapies for PTSD fall into three categories, explains

Young (1995, 177–179). The first is behavior therapy, which aims to reduce the patient's anxiety by deconditioning and "systematic desensitization." The second is cognitive therapy, which aims to provide the patient skills for controlling anxiety, anger, and other negative emotional state. The third is psychodynamic therapy, which works with the patient to understand the meanings of the memories of the traumatic event and to take away the power of the disturbing memories through that analysis (A. Young, 1995, 177–79). These three therapeutic approaches, of course, have been designed and modified through the years for use in sessions months and years after the traumatic event(s).

The second and third of these—cognitive therapy and psychodynamic therapy—really are therapies for the therapist's office and have no parallel with the "folk therapies" in the field. Cognitive processing therapy (CPT), for example, is a common therapy approved by the VA and it is geared toward giving the patient tools for adapting his or her reactions to situations that trigger memories and other symptoms of PTSD. Clearly, CPT needs the therapeutic distance in time and space from the traumatic event and would have no parallel in the short term in the combat zone. The pharmacological therapy does have folk parallels to the degree that warriors use drugs, when they are available, to numb them in the wake of stressful events. Warriors in Vietnam had a lot of drugs easily available to them; warriors in the Middle East have a harder time getting drugs. So we bypass these therapies to hone in on the one we think is most like the folk therapies warriors discover and rely up in the field.

"Behavior therapy" has many variants, but the most common is PET. As David Morris (2015a, 176–77) describes the PET he tried to treat the symptoms of PTSD he experienced having survived an improvised explosive device (IED) blast when he was travelling with a platoon of Marines as a journalist, PET has two components. "Imaginals," the first step, involves the patient's recounting a number of times and in detail the traumatic event, in Morris's case the IED explosion. The second component of PET, "in vivos," asks the patient "to do things in the real world that in some way resembled the traumatic event in question." With both components, explains, Morris, "the governing principle was uncoupling the fear response that had been created by the event from another stimulus" (Morris 2015a, 177).

PET is a member of a class of PTSD therapies called "flooding," an approach created in 1967 by Thomas Stampfl and uses classical learning theory to desensitize the patient, exposing him or her to "a concentrated dose of a frightening stimulus" (D. Morris 2015a, 184). In 1982, as Morris tells us, therapist Terry Keane experimented with "a directed reminiscence technique called 'flooding the imagination' or 'imaginals' to reactivate and, in some way, modify the traumatic memories of Vietnam veterans" (D. Morris 2015a, 184–85). PET is still high on the list of "evidence-based" therapies the Veterans Administration approves for treatment of PTSD in veterans, sometimes even calling PET the "gold standard" treatment for PTSD.

PET and other "flooding" approaches are not without their critics in the scientific community. Morris recounts his own unsuccessful and unpleasant experience with PET, and he summarizes in both his book and a *Slate* essay (D. Morris 2015b) the profession's critique of PET, including the fact that in some cases PET has worsened the PTSD symptoms experienced by the patients in therapy.

The folk therapies in the combat zone we discuss in the following chapters resemble the flooding behavior therapies used by professionals, an approach aimed at "deconditioning" through systematic desensitization, an approach in which the therapist assists the patient's repeated recreation of the heightened state of excitement he experienced in the traumatic event or prolonged stress (A. Young 1995, 177). The patient reaches that state of arousal and then is neither wounded nor killed. The five folk solutions to combat zone stress we examine below reproduce to some extent the state of physiological and mental arousal the warrior experienced hours earlier, and (like the professional behavioral therapy) has value to the warrior because he reexperiences the excitement in a "safe" frame, repeatedly going through that arousal without dire consequences.

We must consider Morris's critique of PET, however, if we are to pursue our fundamental hunch that the folk therapies we discuss in subsequent chapters actually reproduce the processes of flooding therapies.

First, we consider the folk therapies we explore here a sort of battlefield first aid to relieve in the short term the symptoms of PTSD that arise soon after the traumatic event, just as battlefield first aid measures aim to help the wounded warrior until he or she can received professional medical care. We understand that those who return home with some level of symptoms of PTSD will, with luck, receive professional therapy. In a way, then, the efficacy of one professional therapeutic approach or another matters little if the "first aid" that folk therapies offer actually help the warrior cope with stress and its related symptoms in close proximity in time and space to the stressful event of circumstances.

Second, the warriors discover the folk therapies we consider here by trial and error, finding activities that help them. So we follow the warriors in judging the efficacy of their folk therapies. Warriors returning from missions commonly watch movies and listen to music to wind down, but when they engage in the folk therapies we discuss here they often experience the "flooding" characteristic of PET.

Thus, without in any way challenging Morris's critique of the therapies he tried and analyzes, we remain convinced that the folk therapies discovered by the warriors themselves work for them or would be abandoned. Actually, Morris's point and ours are not mutually exclusive—both can be true.

Before moving on to the folk therapies, we should pause briefly to discuss PTSD among female warriors and veterans. The latest estimate is that 11 percent of the veterans from the wars in Iraq and Afghanistan are women, a percentage growing as more and more women are serving there (US Department of Veteran Affairs 2019). Women in those theaters of war were involved in actual combat even before the policy changed to incorporate them into all combat roles, so they are as subject to PTSD as are the male warriors. In addition, several women (and a few men) have experienced sexual assault resulting in what the VA calls MST, military sexual trauma, especially distressing because the perpetrators of the sexual assault are the comrades who are supposed to be part of the "band of brothers and sisters." Women suffer PTSD at rates greater than the men. McLay also reminds us that childhood traumas, such as sexual abuse, are more common in women than in men, and have consequences for reactions to the trauma experienced in the combat zone (2012, 95).

Professional therapies for female veterans tend to be the same as for men—primarily PET and cognitive behavioral therapy (CBT). In the chapters that follow we speculate some on what a particular folk therapy might do for a female warrior, but these are just guesses based on little evidence. As we mentioned in chapter 1, the military is a masculine institution, and the informal folk culture we find there is the culture of the male friendship group. As the patterns of female friendship and play moved toward the patterns in male friendship groups in the 1980s and 1990s, women entering the military seem to be more comfortable in joining and understanding folk groups still based on male friendship. As we argued earlier, Title IX and other forces for female equality gave increasing numbers of women the secret decoder ring for understanding young men. Among other things, women increasingly understand the role of "stylized aggression" in the friendship group, and in joking and pranking and verbal playfighting they often can give as well as get. At the same time, some men will use the play frame to "mask" other motives. Not everyone in the play frame is there voluntarily; not everyone in the play frame has the same power.

Until we have more reliable ethnographic evidence or personal testimony from women, it is difficult to make generalizations about the participation by women warriors in the folk performances of the men. Sure, female warriors probably take the same pleasure in adopting animals in the combat zone as do the men, but do women warriors also sometimes engage in deep play, such as the collection of the body parts of slain enemy warriors? We simply do not know. The available evidence is so heavily skewed toward men that we try to tread lightly in making any claims about the efficacy of folklore in the combat zone for helping women deal with the stress and trauma.

This brief discussion of the biology of stress and trauma, and of professional therapies developed to treat PTSD, prepares us now to examine the five genres of folklore we believe warriors have discovered by trial-and-error to provide some relief from the stress and trauma of living, working, and fighting in the combat zone. Each genre has its own chapter: companion animals, playfighting, video game play, masturbation, and dark, deep play.

II

Folklore Genres

THREE

Animal Companions

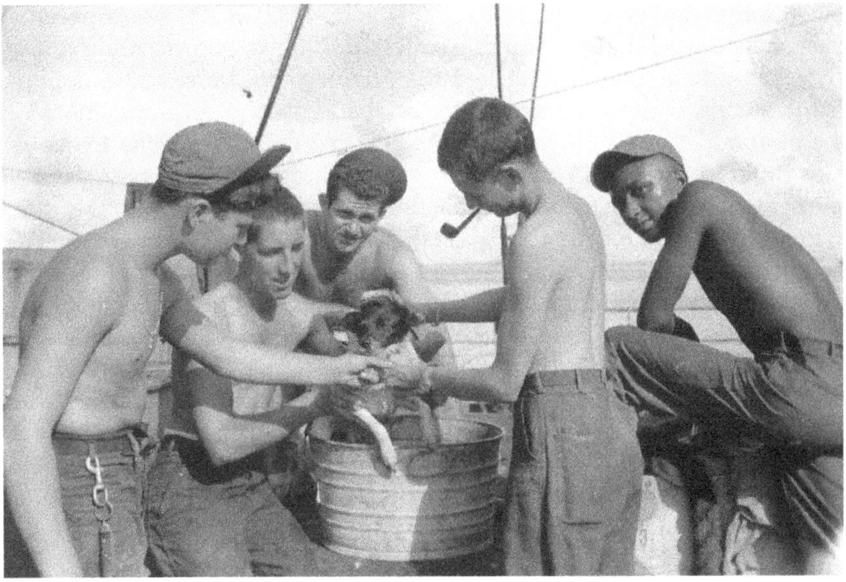

Figure 3.1. Soldiers wash dog, Vietnam. Mechling collection.

The photographic record of the everyday lives of warriors in the combat zone testifies to the presence of animals adopted by the group for distraction and comfort. For centuries sailors have kept cats on board ships to help control the mice and rats, and from the hundreds of vintage military snapshots in Mechling's collection (Mechling 2012), warriors pose for pictures with a range of animals, including parrots, kangaroos, and monkeys aside from the expected dogs and cats. Although some of these animals in the military snapshots are wild animals and their "pet" potential is limited, the cats and dogs adopted aboard ships and by soldiers and Marines in the combat zone fulfill the need humans (and especially Americans) have to keep pets (Grier 2006).

Warriors adopt animals to relieve themselves, even temporarily, of the symptoms of stress caused by living, working, and fighting in the combat zone. Keeping pets serves all sorts of positive functions for physical and mental health, as we shall see, but we also feel comfortable calling pet-keeping a folk custom. Folklorists were slow to come around to considering the human-pet dyad a folk group and the interactions (especially play) between a human and a dog as folk traditions, but Mechling (1989) and then others have demolished the line between human and nonhuman animals to appreciate fully the social and psychological functions of the human/pet dyad. Of course, one thing that makes the military examples different is the collective nature of the human side of the relationship, as groups much larger than the average family adopt the dog. Whole ship companies adopt the cat, just as whole platoons often adopt a dog. This spreads the social and psychological benefits of pet-keeping across a number of humans, and with the dog as the center of care-taking attention, the dog becomes the occasion for the bonding of the humans.

Arluke and Rolfe (2013) devote an entire chapter in their book, *The Photographed Cat*, to "Cats as Shipboard Mascots," and they "read" the photographs to discover sentimentality signs. Entire websites are devoted to photographs of cats on board ships. And dogs adopted in the combat zone show up in a range of published photographs.

MILITARY DOGS IN THE COMBAT ZONE

The relationship between the dog and the warrior illustrates perfectly our argument that folklore and folk customs can provide short-term therapy in the combat zone for the stress warriors experience living, working, and fighting in the combat zone (Cohen 2011). Psychologists and therapists working with PTSD in veterans have found that companion service dogs can do much to lessen the symptoms of PTSD, especially severe PTSD. We shall show here what the psychologists understand about these service dogs in treatment, paying some attention to the effects of a companion dog on the brain and especially the physiology involved with the "fight or flight" response. We then show that there is some evidence, anecdotal by necessity, that dogs can serve the same informal therapeutic functions in the combat zone. As we shall see, that benefit raises military policy questions as adopting pets on deployment is against general orders, and the fate of the adopted dog can exacerbate the symptoms of PTSD.

DOGS AND FORMAL THERAPY FOR PTSD

The Veterans Administration (US Department of Defense) has a National Center for PTSD that keeps track of the variety of treatments for PTSD and the efficacy of those treatments. As we saw earlier, at present CPT and PET are the prevailing therapies for addressing PTSD in veterans, but evidence shows that for some veterans there is a need for additional effective therapies (Stern et al. 2013, 569). The National Center for PTSD favors evidence-based therapies and medications. It does not yet see enough research on the use of dogs in PTSD treatment to fully endorse that therapy. Still, the website for the National Center recognizes the research that shows the general calming, de-stressing effects of dogs as companion animals (see below). Anecdotal evidence suggests that veterans with moderate-to-severe PTSD can benefit from specially trained companion dogs. The self-reports by the thirty-five veterans in Stern et al.'s (2013) study testified that with a companion dog "they experienced improvement in a variety of symptoms, including feeling calmer, less lonely, less depressed, less worried about their own and family's safety, less irritable, and better about themselves as a person" (574).

Iraq veteran Robert Soliz was featured in Colin's (2012) article in *Smithsonian* online about the use of companion dogs as part of the treatment for PTSD. Soliz was suffering the fear, anxiety, depression, and emotional withdrawal common in PTSD sufferers when he was included in "one of four experimental programs nationwide that pair veterans afflicted by PTSD with Labrador and golden retrievers" (Colin 2012). That program, called Paws for Purple Hearts, was founded by social worker Rick Yount in 2008. Another program, Warrior Canine Connection, is based in Baltimore and also has observed the calming influences of the trained PTSD therapy dogs (Colin 2012). As of the 2012 article, about three hundred veterans of Iraq and Afghanistan have participated in the programs, and Mechling witnessed a similar program, The Pathway Home, at the VA hospital in Yountville, California (see Montalván and Witten 2011 for a personal story about how a companion dog was his salvation from PTSD).

Ramakers' (2017) timeline of the history of service and therapy dogs claims that the first use of therapy dogs to help calm patients in a psychiatric ward was in 1919, and she notes that in 1945 the Humane Association "opened and began using Therapy Dogs to help veterans returning from WWII with PTSD," although the condition was known then as "combat fatigue."

Vitztum and Urbanik (2016) point to Boris Levinson (1969) as the beginning of the serious study of human-animal interaction (HAI) and the positive effects of dogs on human health, both physical and mental. HAI studies include the companion animal bond (CAB), animal-assisted activity (AAA), and animal-assisted therapy (AAT), and it is the third field that interests us most as we consider the care for animals as short-term therapy for stress in the combat zone (Vitzum and Urbanik 2016, 173).

Companion dogs help relieve stress in two related ways. First, dogs give their human companions unqualified affection, and the care and feeding dogs require from their humans serves as a distraction from other worries. Rockett and Carr (2014) tackle the ways "attachment theory," popular in human psychology, provides a perspective for understanding the nature of the human-animal bond. From infancy, humans develop attachments to caregivers and those attachments (or their lack) provide the infant and child with "an attachment system" the child invokes in stressful situations. The infant's "innate attachment system" responds to stress, fear, fatigue, or illness (416). People carry this mechanism into adulthood, and the individual's early experiences with attachment figures (e.g., caretakers) help determine later attachments (417).

Beginning with the obvious observation that humans form strong attachments to animal companions, the authors (418) draw upon research on human attachments to outline the elements of the human-animal bond:

> Attachment figures should be (a) dependable sources of comfort (a secure base), (b) sought in times of genuine distress (a safe haven), (c) have their physical presence result in enjoyment and a sense of safety (proximity maintenance), and (d) have their physical absence illicit [*sic*] a sense of distress (separation distress) (418).

Researchers of HAI satisfy themselves that animal companions meet these criteria. Dog owners often referred to their dogs as "safe havens" in this research (419). In reviewing "the pet effect"—that is, "physiological calming in the presence of canines"—Wheeler and Faulkner (2015) report on research showing that boys with insecure-disorganized attachment experienced the calming effects of petting and stroking dogs (427). In fact, as measured by the level of stress-related salivary cortisol samples, petting the dogs lowered the boys' stress level.

We want to pause here to make a few observations about the usefulness of attachment theory in thinking about how the male warriors manage their male friendships and the stress of living, working, and fighting in the combat zone. When young men get to basic training, they have a range of experiences with attachment to other men. Some of this is determined by their relationships with their fathers, brothers, male relatives, and even with male teachers, coaches, scoutmasters, youth group leaders, and the like. The hothouse of basic training, with an agenda of socializing the recruit under conditions reproducing the primary socialization in childhood, makes attachment to the DI and to fellow recruits an issue. The psychologists who study attachment theory tell us that trust is a key element in healthy attachments. Basic training emphasizes trust, putting the recruits through exercises aimed at building trust in the band of brothers. The recruit learns to trust officers (father-figures) and learns to trust his fellow recruits (brothers). These relationships depend on reciprocity of trust.

The warrior in the combat zone absolutely comes to trust his superiors and fellow warriors. Junger, in his book, *War* (2010), his journalistic account of the time he and war photographer Tim Hetherington spent at Restrepo, a remote and dangerous outpost in Afghanistan, says that all time e was not afraid to die; rather, his greatest fear was that he would "fuck up" somehow and get someone else killed. It is a common view among warriors that each fights for the others around him.

One problem facing the warrior in the combat zone is the damage war does to basic trust. The warriors continue trusting each other—they must, and if that trust is broken or violated the consequences are severe. Time and again the testimony in the war memoirs we have read comment on how the experiences in Vietnam, Iraq, and Afghanistan damage one's view of human nature. One trusts his buddies, but he comes to suspect everyone else, sometimes for good reason.

What dogs adopted in the combat zone do is offer the stressed warrior another living being that can be trusted, and the trust between the human and the animal is reciprocal and deep. Animals, especially dogs, are honest in their emotions, and that is something warriors value in a world drenched in deceptions.

Smithson (2009) devotes an entire chapter to "pets" during his deployment in Iraq, and his comments on the platoon's pet bird and adopted dog offer yet another benefit of these animal companions. "These animals," he writes, "give us perspective. They show us resilience and understanding. They show us reality, that we have no control over our situation" (197).

Attachment theory provides a psychosocial explanation for how and why pet animals reduce stress, but the psychophysiological reactions during HAI make clear the hormonal basis for the physical and mental health benefits. Beetz and her colleagues (2012) surveyed sixty-nine original studies on HAI, including studies on animal-assisted interventions (AAI) and animal-assisted therapy (AAT). After reviewing the psychosocial benefits of HAI, Beetz and her colleagues mined the studies for evidence of the hormonal reactions in the brain and mind in response to caring for and stroking pet animals, especially dogs. The studies they surveyed "provide direct evidence that interaction with a friendly companion animal, in particular a dog, positively affects endocrine responses as indicated by changes in the levels of cortisol, epinephrine and norepinephrine, suggesting an attenuation of stress responses via HAI" (Beetz et al. 2012, 6). Beetz and her colleagues argue that "the oxytocin system" is largely responsible for the stress-relief experienced in HAI. "The peptide hormone oxytocin (OT) is produced by the hypothalamus and released into the circulatory system and the brain in response to sensory stimulation" like breast-feeding, sex, touch, and stroking, "usually in the context of trusting relationships" (Beetz et al. 2012, 13). Meg Daley Olmert, who works with the Warrior Canine Connection, also mentions the oxytocin effects in Colin's (2012) *Smithsonian* story.

Given the psychosocial and psychophysiological dynamics in stress relief in HAI, we are not surprised that warriors in the combat zone frequently adopt stray dogs (Taylor, Pooley, and Edwards 2015). Pannella (2010) discusses the antistress benefits of companion dogs and draws upon some veterans' memoirs to show those benefits in detail. Her goal as a lawyer, though, is to argue for a change in the General Orders, which currently prohibit the adoption of stray animals (mainly dogs). General Order 1-A (GO-1A) prohibits pet-keeping and those who violate that order are subject to article 92, failure to obey an order (Pannella 2010, 514). General Order 1B (GO-1B), which superseded GO-1A in 2006, "prevents soldiers from '[a]dopting as pets or mascots, caring for, or feeding any type of domestic or wild animal'" (Pannella 2010, 515).

She then goes on to outline a detailed argument, based on the property rights of warriors, in favor of revising GO-1B(2)(j) "to allow soldiers to care for and possess domestic stray animals for not only legal, but public policy reasons" (Pannella 2010, 516). Pannella notes that the adopted strays provide the immediate stress-relief in the combat zone, and some officers complicate the legal situation by "looking the other way" when warriors in their units adopt strays (2010, 519).

The stress-relieving benefits of the adoptions reach a crisis when the warrior is scheduled to return home. The only options are to release the dog or cat back into the world of strays in the combat zone or, worse yet, to destroy the animal; both options reignite stress in the warrior. At present an expensive option is in operation, as private organizations (like Baghdad Pups) send civilians to Iraq or Afghanistan to rescue the animal, bring it back home, and keep it for the warrior who adopted the animal. This is expensive, though, and out of the reach of most warriors. The solution, argues Pennella, is to modify GO-1B to include stray dogs and cats as permissible "war trophy souvenirs and tourist souvenirs," as currently allowed (2010, 519).

The irony, as Pannella (2010, 531) observes, is that the Department of Defense began research on "animal facilitative therapy to treat PTSD" in

2008, and (as we noted earlier) including companion dogs in the treatment for more severe cases of PTSD has been common therapeutic practice for many years. Warriors in the combat zone discovered the stress-reduction facilitated by adopted cats and animals long ago; only now is professional therapy catching up with the folk therapy.

MILITARY DOGS IN THE COMBAT ZONE

The US military in the current wars in the Middle East uses dogs as part of the operations, including work as sentries, as explosive detectors, as trackers, and in some cases in the search for the wounded and dead. Lemish's (1996) history of "war dogs" recounts centuries of armies using dogs. By the time of the Civil War both armies were using dogs as sentries, but it was in WWI that both sides used dogs as "ambulance assistants" (including finding the wounded on the battlefield and dragging them back behind the lines), as messengers, and as sentries (Lemish 1996, 8–23). In WWII the Coast Guard used dogs in beach patrols from 1942 on, and dogs were used in both the European and Pacific theaters (Lemish 1996, 49, 98–148; Putney 2001). The US Army and Marine Corps used dogs during the Vietnam War (Burnham 2008; Lemish 2009). The military dogs in the Gulf War and the wars in Iraq and Afghanistan served the same rage of functions, from sentries to explosive detection.

In all of these wars, of course, the dog handlers developed close relationships with their dogs, and we assume that for those handlers, the dogs provided mental and physical health benefits. Even military dogs and their handlers, though, face the same dilemma when it is time for the handler to return home. Burnham's (2008) memoir as a handler in the Vietnam War first tells of his harrowing first week as an infantryman and then tells the stories of the succession of war dogs (sentries) he handles for the rest of his tour. Four thousand military dogs were used in the Vietnam War, but the military considered them "expendable equipment" to be left behind when the handlers went home (xi–xii). Military dog handlers faced the same problem as the warriors who adopted dogs in the combat zone. The attachment to the dog helped alleviate the stress in many ways, but the impending abandonment or even killing of the companion dog threatened to rekindle the PTSD the warrior was experiencing. Just as organizations in the United States mobilized to bring home the adopted dogs, so the War Dogs Association, Inc., created by Ron Aiello, worked to bring home the military dogs and created the War Dog Memorial (Burnham 2008, 253).

Lemish (2009) provides a detailed account of the use of military dogs in Vietnam, including the efforts to bring the military dogs home. He also mentions the War Dog Memorial in Bristol Township, Pennsylvania, and the Marine dog memorial in the District of Columbia (228–50). A 2017 theatrical film, *Megan Leavey*, is based on the true story of a female Marine who was a dog handler.

PATCHES AND FRIENDS

So far we have relied on scientific, therapeutic, and even legal expertise to make the case for considering the adoption of pet animals as a form of folk therapy for the stress of warriors' living, working, and fighting in the combat zone. We want to return this discussion to the real lives of the warriors and their adopted pets, and for that we look to the memoirs and accounts by historians and journalists about the actual role of cats and dogs in the everyday lives of warriors.

As Panella (2010) makes clear, stray dogs adopted in the combat zone allay the stress on warriors, offering the warriors distractions, giving them something to care for and care about in the midst of death and destruction. Just having a dog to play with, stroke, and even snuggle with has a strong physiological effect of the warrior's endocrine system. At the same time, Penella shows how current General Orders can add significantly to the stress warriors experience when they must abandon the adopted dog or, worse, euthanize the dog because GO-1B stands in

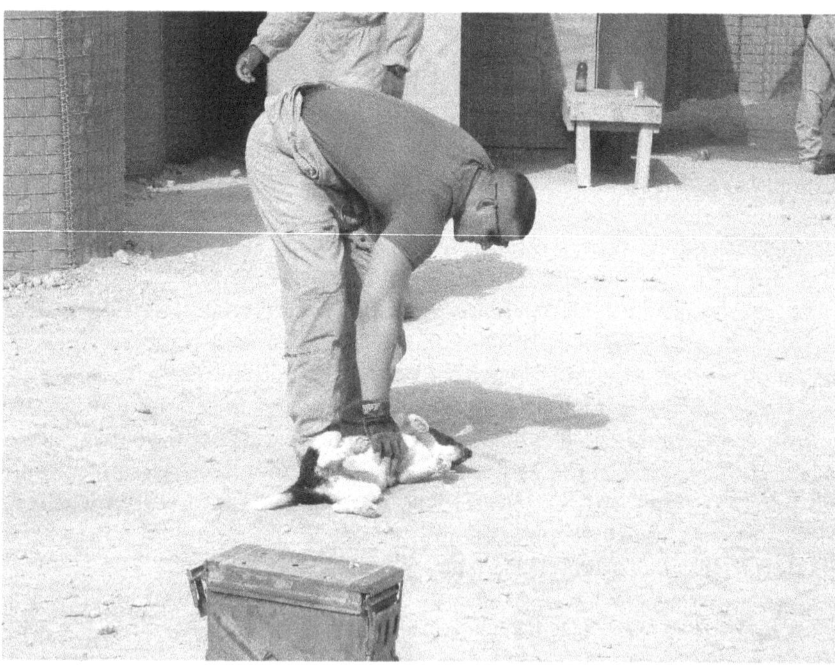

Figure 3.2. Patches. Wallis collection.

the way of the warriors' bringing the adopted dog back home to the United States. Experiencing the loss of the adopted animal, notes Panella (2010, 529), can renew the PTSD that the pet was supposed to ameliorate. "Sometimes," she writes, "even the thought of losing a pet can trigger anxiety or stress that leads to PTSD" (Panella 2010, 530).

We close this chapter with some of the accounts by veterans about their experiences adopting dogs in the combat zone, accounts that add texture to the amazing attachments between the warriors and the adopted dogs. Wallis has his own story to tell, but first we will look at some of the published stories about warriors and their dogs.

The best known account is by Lt. Col. Jay Koppelman (Koppelman and Roth 2006), an account Pannella relies on. Koppelman was with the First Battalion, Third Marines, in Iraq in 2004–2005, a unit that called themselves "the Lava Dogs" (having trained in Hawaii—their variation on "Devil Dogs"). They adopted a stray puppy, which they named "Lava," and over the weeks Koppelman became attached to Lava. His experience and those of his comrades confirmed the literature on the benefits of dog companionship for warriors enduring stress in the combat zone. Koppelman tells some of the horrifying sights he witnessed, from having a Marine's head explode as he was talking with him (2006, 50) to watching stray dogs eating dead bodies (2006, 43). (In fact, several war memoirs from Iraq and Afghanistan report the stomach-turning sights of feral dogs licking up blood and gnawing on dead bodies in the combat zone.)

Cute, frisky, mischievous Lava provided lots of distraction and stress-reduction for Koppelman and his men, but as a senior officer it weighed on his mind that GO-1A forbade the adoption of animals on deployment. He also knew that the Department of Defense had hired private contractors to kill any non-military dogs on the bases (Koppelman and Roth 2006, 56). The more Koppelman thought about how he would have to abandon or even euthanize Lava when it was time for him to return to the United States, the more he knew he had to find a way to get Lava back home. The book chronicles in detail the required machinations and expense, but Lava finally received his shots and was brought to the United States. It was stories like Koppelman's that prompted Pannella's 2010 legal argument to change GO-1B, and it was stories like Koppelman's that led to interventions and assistance by groups like Paws for Purple Hearts and Warrior Canine Connection.

Sulllivan's *Saving Cinnamon* (2009) tells a story similar to Koppelman's but with a more complicated and tense ending. Sullivan tells the story of her brother, Mark, called up from the reserves and sent to Afghanistan, who writes back to his sister about Cinnamon, a puppy adopted by the platoon. Ten to twelve members of the platoon took care of her, and he reported the now-familiar effect the puppy had on the morale of the men. "Cinnamon was a morale booster," writes Christine Sullivan. "A distraction. A piece of home, fun and entertaining. She brightened everyone's day the moment she showed up. Being with her slowed down the fast tempo imposed by a 24/7 military environment. Cinnamon would make you forget where you were just by wagging her tail and by playing chase or by sharing the affection you otherwise couldn't in a war zone" (Sullivan 2009, 35–36). As in other cases, Mark cannot bear the fact that he will have to leave Cinnamon behind or, worse, euthanize her when he is due to return to the States. After lots of arrangement, a dog handler agrees to bring Cinnamon home to Mark, but the handler loses (or abandons her) in Turkey and after a long search Christine finds her and brings her home. Happy ending, but not for many other dogs adopted in the combat zone.

Parnell (2012) offers his own story about how his platoon adopted stray dogs, in Afghanistan, observing that the dogs offered a "small connection to life back home" (2012, 257). And, as in others stories, Parnell reports the distress of his colleagues when someone killed all the dogs (2012, 284).

Here, now, is Wallis's own story of Patches.

I'm not sure who brought Patches back to Expeditionary Patrol Base Hassa. I think it was a PFC [Private First Class] or LCpl [Lance Corporal] from one of the line platoons who went to the little town of Hassa on the southern bank of what we called the "shark's fin" of the Euphrates. Hassa was a small town that seemed to have plenty of dogs. Someone in our company decided that my platoon should do an early morning patrol, inserting into the town before dawn and setting up an observation post, in the hopes that we would have put ourselves in position without any of the townspeople knowing we were there. This was absurd because as soon as we dismounted from our extremely loud turbo diesel-powered vehicles, we could hear the dogs barking at us, despite being a few clicks out of town. You get the idea, there were lots of dogs, and lots of puppies. So Patches showed up at EPB Hassa one day, and we all adopted her as our own.

I'm not sure who gave Patches her name, but that likely doesn't matter, as the origin of her name is self-evident, as surely as a Dalmatian named Spot would be. We loved Patches, well most of us did, because Patches didn't like dark-green Marines. Unfortunately for Patches, our first sergeant was black, and his tent was just around the corner from where Patches slept on an already tiny little outpost for a company of about 125 Marines and sailors. We would be simultaneously delighted and worried each time we hear Patches barking at the 1st sgt or another Marine because she was so cute and harmless.

What I can tell you about Patches is that she and one of the mortarmen in my platoon shared the same name. His name wasn't actually Patches, but Daniel Travino has a random patch of body hair to one side of his lower back, so naturally we called him Patches too.

My wife Julia and I had been dating for less than six months when I deployed that first time, but she was great, sending letters and care packages like it was her job. When she found out about Patches she included items for her too. Julia sent Patches a desert-camouflaged collar with a name tag. I feel like once you put a collar on a dog with a custom name tag, they are a pet and not just a stray animal hanging around.

Stray dogs as pets are not authorized, but because we were alone as a company at Hassa, Patches was allowed to stay, but there were grumblings. Our time at EPB Hassa was relatively short-lived, as we prepared the outpost to turn over to an Iraqi Army unit. We were headed for a larger base where the rest of our company and a few other units were located, just a few miles downriver outside of the small city of Rawah on the northern bank of the Euphrates.

My platoon was the last to leave the EPB before the handover to the Iraqi units and with so much going on, I don't remember thinking much about future accommodations for Patches, but she had left with the rest of the company when they left for our new home near Rawah. After we got to Rawah, we realized Patches wasn't there. Sadly, I think we forgot about Patches in the chaos of the move, but we had a lot going on. Because we had never heard anything come down from our command about getting rid of her, I guess the assumption was that she had gone back to life as a stray. Years later Patches would become a topic for conversation as we tried to figure out what had happened to her. The rumor (a rumor that I carried without recalling my source) was that the maintenance chief in headquarters platoon had thrown her from a moving LAV as the company drove down the highway to Rawah. What a piece of shit (Corps talk for "not a nice person").

The idea that Patches might have been better off, or at least lived longer, had we not taken her in as a puppy is one that cuts pretty close for me. There were several points while we were deployed, and many more since then, that I got the feeling or had the thought "this country and its people would be better off if we never came here." That feeling came up a lot, whether it was confiscating outboard motors from fishermen in villages along the Euphrates before Ramadan, or hearing the wails from family members when we had to detain their husband, father, or son for having a weapon or even a component of a weapon that they shouldn't. Lots of shades of grey, and very few well-defined bad guys to be found.

With Patches that feeling might be even worse. Not to put the life of a puppy above that of Iraqi civilians, but we took Patches in, accepted responsibility for her life, made an emotional connection (she was "our dog") in the way that a family dog would be in America. We may not have known that we would leave EPB Hassa, and have to face the "what now" for Patches, but surely we should have known that we couldn't keep her at Rawah. We knew we weren't supposed to have her in the first place. But the allure of having something innocent and sweet, a reminder of home and our not so distant childhood was too easy to embrace. We named her, and played with her, fed her, and got her a collar. And we were responsible for what was most likely a really shitty way to die.

That's what makes stories of service members and veterans reunited with strays that they adopted as pets on deployment so remarkable: they weren't allowed to have the animal in the first place, and now the dog is in the United States. We can't even get interpreters and their families through the VISA process without putting their lives at risk, waiting years to see whether our enemies get to them first. I'm talking about loyal and brave human beings who were employed by our country to help us fight our wars. So if they have a tough time, the rate of good outcomes for unauthorized pets is depressing. In either instance, such abandonment is not just a mark on our integrity and honor, but bears an emotional and psychological burden.

FOUR

Rough-and-Tumble Playfighting

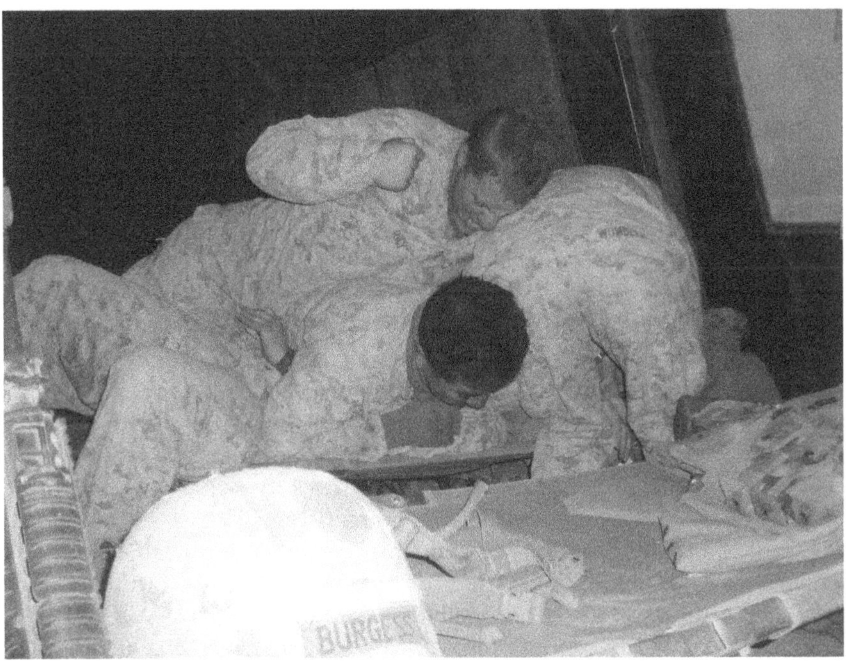

Figure 4.1. Marines in Iraq playfighting. Wallis collection.

The bulk of this chapter was published in the journal *Western Folklore* (vol. 74, 2015, nos. 3 and 4, 275–308) and is reprinted here with permission. Although the authors wrote the original article as a free -standing analysis of the puzzling phenomenon of rough-and-tumble playfighting in the combat zone, the published article (edited slightly here) closes with the point that warrants its inclusion as a chapter in this book—namely that playfighting is a form of folk therapy for addressing the everyday and extraordinary stress of living, working, and fighting in the combat zone.

DEVIL DOGS AND DOG PILES

Whoever designed the dust jacket for journalist Sebastian Junger's 2010 book, *War*, selected for the rear of the jacket a color photograph of the Second Platoon, B Company, engaged in a free-for-all playfight, among the soldiers—some shirtless—grappling with each other in a small space at Outpost Restrepo, a remote outpost in the Korengal Valley in Eastern Afghanistan. Junger was an embedded journalist on assignment from *Vanity Fair* magazine from June 2007 to June 2008. With Junger was war photographer Tim Hetherington, who was killed in Libya in April of 2011. Junger was writing about the experience of combat at that very tenuous outpost and Hetherington was taking both still photographs and video. Hetherington's photographs resulted in a book, *Infidel* (2010), and Hetherington and Junger fashioned a striking, award-winning documentary film, *Restrepo* (2010) from the video footage. Hetherington's photograph of the free-for-all (2010, 127), the one probably chosen by an editor or book designer for the dust jacket, actually is one of a series of photographs showing some sort of playfighting among the soldiers.

Looking at Hetherington's photographs, contextualized as they are by Junger's *War*, the *Restrepo* documentary, and the commentary by both Hetherington and Junger in *Infidel*, we are struck by two things. First, the playfighting is pervasive, which is not surprising, given the ubiquitous presence of playfighting in the friendship groups of male children, adolescents, and adults. Playfighting in a very dangerous combat zone, though, does pose some puzzles, which we address shortly.

Second, Hetherington's photographs of the Marines at Outpost Restrepo (named for a beloved medic of Second Platoon killed in July of 2007) are unmistakably homoerotic. Hetherington's commentary confirms his intention. "As the deployment wore on," writes Hetherington in a commentary on one photograph, "Bonding" (Hetherington 2010, 86),

> attacks on Outpost Restrepo continued, but I became less interested in photographing combat and more interested in the relationships that existed between the soldiers. . . . After I saw this image ["Bonding"], I thought more about the very male atmosphere that existed up at the

> outpost. I saw that there was a special kind of bonding going on—something forged by the extreme circumstances. A friend of mine's grandfather who fought in World War II had commented, "Only in war is it possible for men to demonstrate their love for one another. It's the only place where society sanctions such behaviours." (Hetherington 2010, 234)

The written and visual record of playfighting among the soldiers posted at Outpost Restrepo document just one extended instance of this genre of male play, as memoirs (e.g., Swofford 2003) and vernacular photographs by the warriors themselves since the Great War (Mechling 2012) pile example upon example and suggest that this "horseplay," this "rough-and-tumble play" (as the scholars of play often call it) is integral to the experience of male warriors.

It is easy enough to dismiss playfighting as trivial, as merely "blowing off steam" (the same metaphor that teachers and parents use when sending unruly kids outside), but we believe that playfighting among male warriors deserves a closer, analytical look. Certainly playfighting among warriors achieves the physical release of energy the steam engine metaphor suggests, but that thin interpretation misses other, more complex and often unconscious, meanings. One of the values of folk play and folk rituals is their indirection, the way they address some basic social and psychological anxieties in individuals and groups displacing (in its psychoanalytic meaning) the anxieties and hiding them in some other seemingly unrelated actions. The important social and psychological work done by playfighting among warriors has, therefore, some therapeutic value to the players, and this fact interests us because we seek a greater understanding of the value of folklore as a resource for warriors' dealing with the short-term and long-term stress of trauma in combat. This makes playfighting far from trivial, and we come back to this therapeutic function at the end of this essay.

We draw here upon memoirs, journalists' accounts, some photographic evidence, and the direct experiences of the first author during and after his tour of duty as a Marine in Iraq in 2007 and again in 2008–09 (Wallis 2012). We examine examples of the playfighting among the American men serving in the military. Doubtless there are cultural differences in the performance of masculinity, and the prevailing theory about the social construction of masculinity tends to assume Western patterns of socialization (Mechling 2005). To highlight the meanings of playfighting among the male warriors, we ask whether female warriors also participate in such playfighting. We look at playfighting in a range of settings, some relatively safe (basic training, downtime even in a combat zone, etc.) and some more dangerous (e.g., at Outpost Restrepo).

ROUGH-AND-TUMBLE PLAY

The warriors at Restrepo were engaged in what play scholars call rough-and-tumble (R&T) play, a form of playfighting. R&T play both fascinated and puzzled scholars from the earliest interest in animal play (Groos 1898). Darwinism gave a boost to animal studies in the late nineteenth century, and animal play—especially playfighting in animals—puzzled scientists (Burghardt 2005). Playfighting seems to have no survival value in natural selection; indeed, playfighting expends precious calories, carries the risk of injury, and draws away attention to potential predators. Yet, mammals play from young ages. At first scientists accounted for R&T play by seeing it as anticipatory socialization, as practice for skills needed as adults. Doubtless play does serve such instrumental functions. But more recently scholars have come to the view that mammals playfight for the expressive pleasure of playing (Sutton-Smith 1997, 29–34).

A good deal of the research on playfighting in humans looks at gender differences. Pellegrini (1988, 1993) argues that playfighting in boys helps develop social competence, and several researchers doing direct observation of playfighting in boys note that the boys tend to use "warrior discourse" (Jarvis 2006, 273; Jordan 1995, 76; O'Donnell and Sharpe 2004) in their R&T play. Scholars directly observing boys' R&T playfighting also note that in an age of children's television, the boys often "script" their play by adopting characters and even plots from television shows. Sutton-Smith's graduate students observed in the 1980s that the children at a Quaker school regularly played Power Rangers (a popular television show then) in their free play (Botvin and Sutton-Smith 1977; Sutton-Smith, Gerstmeyer, and Meckley 1988), and more recently Jarvis (2006, 277) observed primary school boys re-enacting characters and scenes from *Beyblades*, a popular Japanese cartoon show. The television-scripted voluntary play by these boys on the playground thus served many functions, teaching the boys the hierarchy of a male friendship group and the difference between fantasy violence and real violence, a point also made by Jones (2002).

The ability to distinguish between stylized, violent acts in the play frame and violence in "real life" is extremely important and that ability is crucial in the R&T playfighting research that shows that playfighting in youth actually creates "neural pathways" for boys' understanding the play frame of sports and other male competitions (e.g., verbal dueling). Jarvis (2006) and Jones (2002, 37, 116) both note that boys who do not acquire the ability (through playfighting) to distinguish violence in the play frame from violence in everyday life actually become less socially successful and more aggressive as adults.

This too-brief summary of the positive aspects of R&T playfighting in boys helps us see the history the warriors bring to the male friendship group in combat zones. Most have acquired the competence necessary to enter the play frame and to distinguish between stylized violence and real violence. They understand the play frame of the game or contest, and they understand that what happens inside the play frame does not mean what it would mean outside the play frame (Bateson 1972, 183). They understand that the trust involved in entering the frame of the playfight already signals to the other player(s) that they have a close relationship, and they experience the R&T playfighting as a form of intimate connection. But R&T playfighting in a combat zone has important psychological and social work to do that is not always present in R&T playfighting in less dangerous and less stressful places and times.

ROUGH-AND-TUMBLE PLAYFIGHTING IN COMBAT ZONES

Amateur photographs going back to the late nineteenth century, when inexpensive portable cameras and roll film made snapshots a favorite way for ordinary people to preserve memorable moments and experiences, provide ample testimony as to R&T play by boys and men, including soldiers, sailors, and Marines (Bronner 2006; Mechling 2012). Bronner (2012, 114–51) documents and analyzes the "class scraps" and other large-scale playfighting events on American college campuses, also going back to the 19th century. Although some of these events included women, by far the most common and dirtiest (e.g., fighting in mud) scraps are among men. Clearly, male warriors bring to their experience in the military a vast set of experiences with R&T playfighting from childhood and youth.

War memoirs record frequent instances of R&T playfighting, even in combat zones. In his memoir of the first Gulf War, *Jarhead* (2003), Anthony Swofford explains two of these customs in the middle of describing how his unit began misbehaving when a reporter was trying to interview and film them for a story. They are playing a game of touch football, comically wearing their gas masks, when the play slips quickly into a game of tackle. "Combs kicks Kuehn in the ass," writes Swofford,

> and we all jump on the pile, punching each other, and it doesn't matter whom you hurt, because you're not punching hard, you're not punching to hurt, but only to punch. The half-speed fight degenerates into a laughter-filled dog-pile, with guys fighting their way from the bottom to climb back to the top, king of the pile, king of the Desert. We're swearing and shouting and shrieking through our masks. This is fun, plain mindless fun, the kind grunts are best at. (2003, 20)

Swofford then goes on to describe the tradition of the "field fuck,"

> an act wherein marines violate one member of the unit, typically someone who has recently been a jerk or abused rank or acted antisocial, ignoring the unspoken contracts of brotherhood and camaraderie and esprit de corps and the combat family. The victim is held fast in the

> doggie position and his fellow marines take turns from behind. (2003, 20–21)

Swofford reports feeling both frightened and exhilarated by the field-fuck, which is performed fully clothed. "The exhilaration isn't sexual," explains Swofford, "it's communal—a pure surge of passion and violence and shared anger, a pure distillation of our confusion and hope and shared fear" (2003, 21).

Another playfighting custom in the combat zone is "bloodying" or blood in, blood out as described by Junger (2010, 23, 158). A few of Hetherington's photographs (2010, 128–31) record an instance of the platoon's traditional ritual of "bloodying" a comrade on his birthday or on some other transitional event, like going on leave or returning from leave. This ritual—one is reminded of the branding ritual included by Swofford (2003, 50–51) in *Jarhead*—involves a "victim" who is seized, pinned down, and "bloodied" (symbolically, but often literally) by a group of his comrades. Hetherington's photograph of the smiling victim of the sequence affirms the play frame for being "bloodied" and signals for the viewer the male bonding functions of this ritual (Mechling 2008c, 2009).

Wallis (first author) knows this tradition as the birthday beatdown, wherein a platoon or possibly a smaller number of fellow soldiers and Marines administer to "the birthday boy" a "beating" (also Finkel 2009, 117). Wallis experienced one of these during his deployment in Iraq in 2007. Here is the story he tells:

> My birthday was coming up and I knew that the platoon would want to give me a birthday beatdown. But my birthday was the same day as a sergeant everybody disliked, so I figured maybe mine would escape notice. That day I came into the hooch [living shelter] and walked back to my rack [bed], and as I got closer to it I saw on my bed a large sheetcake, you know, the sort they sell in Safeway. How they found a cake out there I'll never know. But there was this cake with a note on it. I picked up and opened the note: "Sorry about the beatdown." I looked up and the whole platoon suddenly was behind and around me. They were all smiling, and the beatdown began [told to Mechling July 10, 2014].

Although the birthday beatdown Wallis received from his friends was rough, not administered full strength but rough nonetheless, Wallis reports enjoying it. It made his birthday perfect. The play frame of the birthday beatdown affirmed that Wallis had close-enough, affectionate-enough relationships with the others that they could engage in the playfighting, that he belonged to the group.

Wallis sees more in the paradoxical pleasures of the beatdown. The beatdown, he explains, "is about pain, and taking delight in pain. Marines wear their pain like a badge of honor." Wallis notes that the "prestige of pain is found throughout grunt culture." The Marines worship pain. Medals awarded for "valor in combat" are most valuable when the valor is displayed while the hero is gravely wounded. Wallis's training company at the Marine Corps' School of Infantry had "Hate and Discontent" as its official motto. When as veterans they get together to tell stories, they show the most nostalgia for the pain. "What matters the most," explains Wallis, "is taking the pain and loving it, taking the pain and turning it against the common enemy, taking the pain so that others don't have to." Energizing the nostalgia for the beatdown is nostalgia for the pain (told to Mechling July 10, 2014).

Seven years later, in law school, Wallis reports (July 10, 2014), he was feeling a bit sad on his birthday, remembering and missing that birthday beatdown in Iraq, when he heard behind him in the halls of the classroom building, "Hey, happy birthday, motherfucker," and another Marine veteran also in law school administered a few punches to Wallis's arm and torso. They laughed together. Wallis says that this mini-beatdown raised his spirits and salvaged a birthday that seemed like just another day in law school.

The birthday beatdown should not be confused with the blanket party, which is not administered in the play frame and which is meant as punishment by the group of a member who gets them all in trouble and brings extra punishment on the group. As depicted in the theatrical films *Full Metal Jacket* (1987) and *A Few Good Men* (1992), those applying the beating in a blanket party attack the victim in his rack, trapping him under the blanket by pulling it tight on the sides and taking turns hitting the victim. In *Full Metal Jacket* the punishers put hard bars of soap in socks and administer the blows with that hard weapon (a practice quite common, according to other accounts). The blanket party is a forbidden practice within the military, and it is hard to tell whether it is common anymore. Contrasting the blanket party with the birthday beatdown, however, affirms the importance of the play frame and its signal about the relationships between the participants.

THE PARADOX OF PLAY

Bateson's remarkable 1972 [orig. 1955] essay, "A Theory of Play and Fantasy," suggests a path for the analysis of the playfighting among male American warriors. It is well-known that in this formulation of the "play frame" Bateson is struck by the paradox of play, that (as he puts it, using animal playfighting as his example) "not only does the playful nip not denote what would be denoted by the bite for which it stands, but, in addition, the bite itself is fictional" (1972 [1955], 182). That's the well-known part. But Bateson then goes on to say that sometimes this paradox has an odd effect, and he uses some examples from action films to show how some images "did not denote that which they seemed to denote, but these same images did really evoke that terror which would have been evoked" by a real event or threat (183). Bateson then turns to some examples of films that encode sexuality. In the 1952 film *Hans Christian Andersen*, writes Bateson (183–84),

> the hero starts out accompanied by a boy. He tries to get a woman, but when he is defeated in this attempt, he returns to the boy. In all of this, there is, of course, no homosexuality, but the choice of these symbolisms is associated in these fantasies with certain characteristic ideas, *e.g.*, about the hopelessness of the heterosexual masculine position when faced with certain sorts of women or with certain sorts of male authority. In sum, the pseudohomosexuality of the fantasy does not stand for any real homosexuality, but does stand for and express attitudes which might accompany a real homosexuality or feed its etiological roots. The symbols do not denote homosexuality, but do denote ideas for which homosexuality is an appropriate symbol.

Bateson's stunning insight here is that play engages "a special combination" of primary (unconscious) and secondary (conscious) processes (185).

Bateson's insight helps us see two different truths about male playfighting. *Playfighting both is and is not combat. Playfighting both is and is not sex*. It looks and feels like combat, and it looks and feels like sex, but the peculiar, paradoxical genius of the playfighting play frame is that it both is and is not either of these.

Although it is tempting to deal separately with the analytical insights that playfighting among real warriors "is and is not real fighting" and "is and is not sex," our first attempt at separating the two paradoxes failed. This is because aggression and sex are intimately related. *Eros* and *Thanatos* embrace in human affairs (Freud 1922 [1920]). So it is with warriors. As Grossman (2009) and others point out, the male physiological response to both aggression and sexual arousal is pretty much the same. The same hormones and the same parts of the brain work in the arousal. One of the veterans quoted by Tick (2005, 124) observed that "I wrestled men to death in hand-to-hand combat. That experience was far more intimate and erotic than sex or love can ever be."

Many of the veterans interviewed by Grossman testified to the sexual excitement of shooting a gun, especially a fully automatic weapon, and they compared "the power and pleasure of explosively spewing a stream of bullets . . . [to] the emotions felt when explosively spewing a stream of semen" (2009, 137). More important for the argument we are developing here is the point Grossman makes in his chapter on "Killing at Sexual Range." Grossman discusses the psychology and physiology of killing at a range of distances from the enemy, beginning with maximum range (artillery, bombing) to "sexual range," the most intimate range of close combat. "Thrusting the sexual appendage (the penis) deep into the body of the victim" in rape, writes Grossman (2009, 137), "can be perversely linked to thrusting the killing appendage (a bayonet or knife) deep into the body of the victim."

In *War* (2010), Junger notes the consequences of the association between violence and sex for these soldiers. "The one absolute impossibility at Restrepo" he writes,

> was sex with a woman, and the one absolute impossibility back home was combat. Whether the men realized it or not, they had made a rough trade where one risked becoming a stand-in for the other. . . . There was so much sexual energy up at Restrepo that it might as well have been a Miami nightclub, except that the only outlet for it was combat, so that's what the men spent their time thinking about. (2010, 151)

The value of playfighting is that the fight is "not real." The combatants do not carry bayonets or knives (pugil stick training is an exception we address below), but the physical aggression in playfighting represents the real aggression that it is performing and provides the same physical and physiological responses as would fighting outside of the play frame. Male high school and college wrestlers sometimes report getting erections while grappling closely with an opponent, an embarrassing and generally rare event, but one that confirms how rough-and-tumble playfighting invokes the responses that link aggression and sex (Delfino and Mechling 2017).

Dundes's (1997) writing on the relations between games and war make explicit how the male playfighting—from informal folk games like Smear the Queer to formal games like American football—resembles male-on-male rape. Playfighting is about power and domination, with the ultimate goal of putting the male opponent "down" (i.e., in the submissive, female position in sex) and penetrating his "endzone" (1997, 27). And although Dundes relies more on the games' structures and the folk speech used by the players, while Grossman looks at the physical, physiological, and psychological experiences of the real fighting, if we combine both insights with Bateson's point about the simultaneity of primary and secondary process in play, we come to understand how warriors' rough-and-tumble playfighting, neither fighting nor having sex, creates the arousal of both.

As Bateson and others (e.g., Handelman 1977; Goffman 1974) note, the play frame is a fragile one, easily broken. Players usually work quickly to repair the frame if they care about the interaction. In male playfighting, a poke too hard, a hold too tight, even a detectable erection can break the frame. Junger saw at Restrepo a soldier who, he thought, had difficulty maintaining the playfight frame. "Bobby claimed a kind of broad-spectrum sexuality," writes Junger,

> that made virtually no distinction between anything, and as the months went by that expressed itself in increasingly weird ways. He would take someone down with a quick headlock and create a kind of prison-yard sense of violation without actually crossing some ultimate line. . . . Ultimately, it made me think that if you deprive men of the company of women for too long, and then turn off the steady adrenaline drip of heavy combat, it may not turn sexual, but it's certainly going to turn weird. (2010, 224)

Junger goes on to chronicle Bobby's "weird" behavior—"strange pantomimed man-rapes" and "smoochy come-ons" (2010, 224). Bobby was not gay, observes Junger,

> but a year on a hilltop somehow made pretending otherwise psychologically necessary. And it wasn't gay anyhow: it was just so hypersexual that gender ceased to matter. Someone once asked Bobby whether, all joking aside, he would actually have sex with a man up here. "Of course," Bobby said. "It would be gay not to." (2010, 225)

Bobby's reasoning was that "real men" need sex, no matter the partner, and that to abstain was less masculine. Some of the other men at Restrepo worried that Bobby and his friend Jones would actually be capable of raping a member of the platoon if they caught someone alone.

Junger's observations about Bobby point to some of the subtleties of the precarious balance between violence and sex in the playfighting of male warriors. As Junger says, it's not that Bobby is gay—Junger believes he is not; Junger wants to call Bobby's behavior "hypersexual," and he attributes that to the special circumstances at Restrepo. Junger also detects in Bobby someone who can't really maintain the play frame in playfighting—he gets dangerously close to breaking the frame and sometimes does.

Junger thought that Bobby was being weird, but maybe Bobby understands the paradox of the play frame better than most. His declaration that "it would be gay not to" have sex with a man at Restrepo reminds us of the folk game gay chicken, in which two players of the same sex move closer and closer towards each other until one of them backs off or they end up kissing; the first person to back off is the "gay chicken." The game embodies the same paradox Bobby announces—namely, it would be gay not to engage in an act in the play frame that would be gay if performed outside of the play frame.

The first author (Wallis) reports that members of his platoon would play gay chicken when bored in their "downtime." The game had special resonance with the Marines because of the importance of "bearing" in the Corps. Recruits are socialized from day one into the notion of bearing, which means "keeping your war-face on" without betraying any emotions or thought behind the hardened mask. In fact, Wallis's platoon invented a bearing game, in which two Marines would face off and use just words to get the opponent to lose his "bearing." When members of the platoon played gay chicken, though, the players could use both words and physical acts. The movement toward each other, trying to break the other's bearing with words and acts, could result in one Marine's kissing another. The participants and audience understood that the kiss did not mean that either player was gay, because (like Junger's example of Bobby) turning away and breaking frame meant that the player feared committing a gay act. In the logic of the game (Bobby's logic, too), the fear of committing a gay act was what exposed the player as gay. To maintain your bearing while playing gay chicken meant that you had no insecurities to betray.

Significantly, both the bearing game and gay chicken were played within the small, high context group—usually a fire-team of three or four Marines, at most a platoon. Sometimes the Marines would use gay chicken to resolve who got some good in limited supply, like a "care package" of goodies from home. Wallis speculates that the game very often was a way for two Marines—close buddies in the small group—to settle minor disputes, where perhaps one person was "butt-hurt" about something and the conviviality of the game would go a long way toward breaking that tension. This is one of the important functions of the play frame, the use of indirection to repair relationships. As Bateson notes, even entering the play frame with another already announces the relationship, because the play frame requires confidence and trust in the other; this is all the more true in the bearing game and in gay chicken.

As we expected, there is yet another use of gay chicken in the male folk group. Bateson's frame analysis assumes the players are in the frame voluntarily, have equal power, and that their motive for entering the contract of the frame is to have fun or to express a relationship. But Goffman (1974) corrected Bateson's romantic view of the frame to remind us that not everyone is in a play frame voluntarily and that some players enter the frame with the selfish manipulation of others in mind, as in the con game. Sutton-Smith and Kelly-Byrne (1984) likewise remind us that people can use play to "mask" motives. We were not surprised to learn from one Marine in Wallis's unit that he saw at least one instance where a player used the gay chicken game to intimidate and shame another Marine, getting the target to leave the room.

Junger attributes the behavior of the men at Restrepo to the absence of women, but if pressed he would probably amend his statement to note that gay and bisexual warriors at Restrepo and elsewhere do not necessarily miss the access to sex with women. For them, consensual sex with other men at the outpost is as inaccessible as consensual sex with women. When the "steady adrenaline drip of heavy combat" is turned off, as Junger puts it, then only masturbation and playfighting serve as satisfactory substitutes. These activities sustain the association of aggressive violence with sex.

BASIC TRAINING

Context is everything, so let us back up a bit and join the male soldier or Marine in basic training to see how everything leads to the playfighting we see in Hetherington's photographs at Restrepo and in the written accounts of playfighting in veterans' memoirs and journalists' accounts.

Basic training seems guaranteed to intensify the link between *eros* and *thanatos*, between the pleasures of violence and the pleasures of sex. Most young men in basic training are experiencing the crescendo of their sexual maturation. At the same time, basic training also takes away from the young men what they have enjoyed since infancy—namely, control over one's basic bodily functions. The male body looms large as fact and symbol in basic training. Father figures control basic bodily functions, from eating and sleeping to shitting and pissing (we use the folk language here—see Mechling 2014). Basic training affords no privacy in these basic bodily functions. The constant surveillance, control of bodily functions by the drill instructors, and total lack of privacy in basic training even suppresses masturbation to the point of extinction, a remarkable achievement, given the sex drive of young men in their late teens and twenties.

Relevant for our understanding of playfighting in combat zones is the basic training in close combat. The irony here is that combat in America's recent wars (since Vietnam) has rarely involved killing at the three closest ranges discussed by Grossman—"killing at edged-weapon range," "killing at hand-to-hand combat range," "and killing at sexual range" (2009, 120–37). Modern weaponry has made obsolete the close combat common in the two World Wars, Korea, and sometimes in Vietnam. Yet, fundamental to basic training in the American military is training in close combat. Our hunch, of course, is that this training has a direct psychological and physical connection to playfighting in the combat zone, even though the skills acquired in basic training are in no realistic sense preparatory for the sort of combat skills the warrior will need on the battlefield. Something else must be at play in this continuing inclusion of and commitment to training in close combat.

Consider, for example, pugil stick training. Recruits look forward to these training sessions because they are a welcome break from the other activities of basic training. Young boys practice unprotected versions of stick fighting all the time, so pugil stick training doubtless stirs memories of that childhood play. In this case, two recruits—typically from different platoons—don protective gear (helmets, neck protection, hockey gloves, and groin protection) and engage in close combat with thick sticks about four feet long and padded at both ends. The combatants face off and, holding their sticks with both hands, attempt to land blows on the opponent to knock him down. Typically their comrades surround the combatants, putatively to learn the offensive and defensive moves they see, but also because the contest pits one platoon against the other, so platoon pride beyond individual pride is at stake.

As we said, although the rationale for including pugil stick training in basic training is that it prepares the warrior for close, hand-to-hand combat with knives (K-bars) or bayonets, the recruits most likely will not be called upon to use these skills. Most of the weapons used in Iraq and Afghanistan, for example, kill at a distance; only rarely will a warrior use close combat skills. So we return to our question—namely, why do the armed services retain pugil stick exercises in basic training?

Pugil stick fighting taps very basic physiological, psychological, and even social drives and motives in the young man. Boys forge their masculinity largely through physical contests with other boys. Playing with sticks turns into swordfights and other forms of male contest with sticks. A sociobiologist might argue that we are seeing in stick dueling boys' anticipatory socialization or, at least, an evolutionary survival. But that explanation ignores the consummatory pleasures the boys enjoy fighting with the sticks. It is fun. Boys fighting with sticks are having fun and recruits fighting with pugil sticks are having fun. Wallis notes that pugil stick exercises are one of the few occasions in basic training for physically touching a live opponent, and the carefully framed rules and safety equipment make a pugil stick contest more fun than the unstructured brawl where the play frame is easily broken as violence escalates.

We also see significance in the sticks. Though our understanding of the pleasures of the pugil stick contest is plenty rich enough by pointing to the pleasures of the contest and the pleasures of physical contact in an institutional setting where that is carefully framed, we see no reason to doubt that the pugil stick stands in for the penis in the contest (see Mechling [2008c] for similar symbolism of the paddle in fraternity hazing). Folk speech equating sticks, knives, swords (another word for condom is "sheath"), and spears with the penis provides plenty of evidence for this view. Goytan (1998) noted in the camp counselor's ritual of pissing out the campfire the folk speech used by the teen boy counselors—they crossed streams and called it dueling. Mechling (2001, 2014) looks to psychoanalytic theory to see dueling with male streams of urine as dueling. And men sometimes actually "duel" or have "swordfights" with their erect penises.

Recall that Dundes argues that the goal of most male contests is to "put down" the opponent, putting him into the submissive, female position in intercourse and to penetrate the opponent's "endzone." The goal in pugil stick fighting is not to penetrate him but to knock him down with your stick, metaphorically to knock down the other male with your symbolic penis.

After basic training the warriors deployed to Iraq and Afghanistan (the populations we know the most about) have faced conditions similar to those in basic training—a lack of privacy for bodily functions, a lack of women for actual heterosexual behavior (excluding impermissible consensual sex with women and rape, a too-common phenomenon), and circumstances in which the paradoxical strength and vulnerability of the male body is demonstrated daily.

The very male folk culture of a platoon, for example, which is still small enough at forty or so to be the effective folk culture for the warrior (who also experiences smaller folk cultures of the eight-to-twelve men in the squad), inundates the individual warrior with stories, jokes, pornographic images, pranks, taunts, and other folk genres keeping sex on these men's minds. This heterosexual male culture (though populated with gay and bisexual men, to be sure) must accomplish a delicate balance. The men must sustain performances of normative male heterosexuality for everyone, including themselves, which necessarily involves the heteronormative repression of the feminine in the self and the denigration of the feminine in other men and in women.

At the same time, the living and fighting circumstances of the squad and the platoon in combat zones lead to an intense bonding between the brother warriors. "Repeatedly," notes Grossman (2009, 89), "we see combat veterans describe the powerful bonds that men forge in combat as stronger than those of husband and wife." Given the strong bonds of affection between male warriors and American cultural norms carefully choreographing one male's touching another, the only way to satisfy the strong human need to be touched and held and stroked in stressful situations is through carefully framed behavior, most notably the R&T play of playfighting.

Lyman's (1987) analysis of "the fraternal bond as a joking relationship" captures well the role of homoerotic play, especially aggressive homoerotic play, as the glue holding together a close male group. Men are capable of real violence and aggression against each other, so to manage those impulses (which threaten the solidarity of the male friendship group), men in groups engage in stylized aggression, from verbal aggression (e.g., ritual exchanges of insults) to informal R&T playfighting to more formal games and sports. In male friendship groups, "intimacy is split from sexuality in order to eroticize the male bond" (Lyman 1987, 175). This move has two consequences based in the need for the "early repression of the son's erotic bond with his mother" (see Chodorow 1978). First, the move serves to make women "sexual objects" and accounts for the misogyny in the folklore of male groups, including the military (C. Burke 2004). Second, the move attaches the excitement of sexuality to rules and rule-breaking in the male group. Lyman turns to Gray's (1959, 89–90) distinction between comradeship and friendship in the male bonding. "Comradeship is based upon an erotic of shared danger," writes Lyman, paraphrasing Gray, "but is based upon the loss of an individual sense of self to a group identity, while friendship is based on an individual's intellectual and emotional affinity to another individual."

The result is this: "In the eros of friendship one's sense of self is heightened; in the eros of comradeship a sense of self is replaced by a sense of group membership." Comradeship brings ecstasy, argues Gray, and a sense of immortality through sacrifice of the individual for the group (1959, 45–46). Thus, misogyny and the eros of male comradeship work together to create the strong bond in male groups.

WOMEN WARRIORS AND R&T PLAYFIGHTING

We focus here on R&T playfighting in the folk cultures of male warriors because (until recently) to talk about American warriors was to talk about men in groups. Women have been involved in war throughout our history, of course (Solaro 2006, 10–11), and female nurses were wounded or killed in service during the Vietnam War. In the Gulf War in 1991, more than forty thousand servicewomen participated in the war, and later that decade President Clinton opened some combat roles to women (Holmstedt 2007, xviii). American servicewomen were in combat in Iraq even before expanded combat roles were open to them. By the time Holmstedt published her book, *Band of Sisters*, in 2007, more than seventy female warriors had been killed and more than four hundred wounded in the war in Iraq (2007, xix). By the spring of 2013, 144 women warriors had been killed and 800 wounded in Afghanistan, Iraq, and Kuwait (Biank 2013, 5).

Although their numbers are still small and most units in the combat zone do not have a critical mass of women in the unit, many servicewomen clearly face the same stressful situations as many servicemen. Some readers might ask, fairly, whether our argument here about the shape and meanings and functions of R&T playfighting in the folk cultures of male friendship groups, especially of warriors in combat zones, applies at all to female warriors.

The short answer is no. We cannot prove the negative, but none of the evidence we have suggests that women warriors in the wars in Iraq and Afghanistan engage in the R&T playfighting we find in the male combat units. Wallis's unit in Iraq had no women, so he has no direct, ethnographic experience with women warriors in basic training or during his time deployed. Moreover, a sample of the memoirs and reporters' accounts of the lives of women warriors in the combat zones in Iraq and Afghanistan (Williams and Staub 2005; Solaro 2006; Holmstedt 2007, 2009; Biank 2013; Thorpe 2014; Lemmon 2015; Hegar 2017) fail to describe anything like the R&T playfighting we find so common in accounts of and by male warriors.

The reasons for this absence in the experience of women warriors are worth a brief look and they confirm the unique role of R&T playfighting in the management of relationships within the male folk group.

Scientific studies of playfighting in mammals find no significant sex differences in the playfighting of the young, but in young humans the sex segregation of play begins early. An ethnographic study of over two hundred preschool children (ages 3–5) in nine Philadelphia area preschools in the 1980s found that almost every instance of playfighting, especially R&T playfighting, involved boys (Sutton-Smith, Gerstmyer, and Meckley 1988). Two excellent ethnographies of the playground play of elementary school children, Thorne's (1993) study of fourth- and fifth-graders in California and Michigan, and Beresin's (2010) study (based on observations in 1991, 1999, and 2004) of third- to fifth-graders in the Philadelphia area give us a snapshot of gender differences as the children age. Thorne (1993, 92) found that in both playgrounds she studied the boys engaged in more R&T playfighting than did the girls, whose main mode of physical interaction between the bodies of the boys and their own were chasing games (1993, 68–71). Occasionally the chasing games ended with some wrestling to the ground, but this was rare (1993, 72). Thorne is careful to avoid the stereotyping of boys' and girls' play, noting (for example) that R&T playfighting is not a dichotomous gender difference and that the "within gender" differences are greater than those between the genders (1993, 104). Both the boys and girls seem to enjoy "borderwork," playing at the boundaries between the gender-segregated play, and she displays special interest in those daring children who "crossed" those borders to engage in the stereotypical play and play groups of the opposite gender.

Beresin's (2010) ethnographic work in an East Coast playground one and then two decades after Thorne's observations found even more crossing or, more accurately, even more integration of boys' and girls' play, especially in the game of Sui, short for Suicide, a game similar to handball and dodgeball (2010, 44–45). Just as Hughes (1993, 1999) found the elementary-age children playing four-square in her extended ethnographic work using the game to manage power relationships within the play group, the children Beresin observed found Sui the perfect game for creating and managing power relationships. Few girls played Sui in 1991, but by Beresin's return to the playground in 1999 the girls commonly played the game by themselves or with boys (2010, 47–8). By her revisit to the playground in 2004, Beresin found that the girls played Sui every day and that they were also playing football and basketball (2010, 121).

The evolution of the physicality of girls' play from what Thorne observed in 1976–1977 to what Beresin observed in 2004 suggests that the gender revolution intended in part by passage of Title IX of the Education Amendments Act of 1972 has been successful, that young women's accessibility to the experiences of team sports has introduced them to the previously very male folk cultures of those sports. Girls' play in the United States has come over the past century to resemble more and more the play of boys, and the ethnographic work by Beresin and others confirm that this trend has accelerated since the passage of Title IX. Increasing numbers of women are participating in competitive high school wrestling, for example, a sport most relevant to this inquiry about R&T playfighting (Lewin 2007; also Delfino and Mechling 2017). Several memoirists and reporters mention the experience of these women warriors as athletes in high school and college, and Solaro (2006, 243–44) explicitly connects the fitness of the women warriors to these athletic experiences and Title IX.

And yet, the accelerating willingness of young women to engage in forms of physical play with each other and with young men does not seem to result in R&T playfigfhting between women warriors or with men. We can speculate on the reasons for this absence.

A primary challenge for men in the combat zone is to prove their manhood (Beneke 1997), always a fragile construction (Mechling 2005), and to perform their masculinity in such a way as to ensure that their genuine, experienced close bonding is understood as "brotherly love" between heterosexual men (even, or maybe especially, for gay and bisexual men). R&T playfighting and associated homoerotic play with the male bodies are crucial in this delicate construction and maintenance of masculinity under stress. The Batesonian paradox of this R&T playfighting for the men is that it both is and is not fighting, both is and is not sex. And, as we have seen, one of the further paradoxes of this homoerotic play is that "it would be gay not to" engage in the play. R&T playfighting uniquely addresses the psychological and social needs of the male warriors.

In contrast, our reading of the memoirs and reporters' accounts of female warriors who have been in combat zones in Iraq and Afghanistan points to a very different set of interpersonal challenges. Feminist psychoanalytic theory, which informs much of our view of the construction, maintenance, and repair of masculinity (Chadorow 1978; Frosh 1994; Mechling 2005), holds that femininity does not need to be "proven" the same way fragile masculinity must be proven by separation from the feminine. Women in the war zones testify that they need to "prove" that they are as competent soldiers as the men (e.g., Lemmon 2015, 58). They do face interpersonal issues of a sort different from those the men deal with through the folklore of the male friendship group. Williams and Staub (2005, 13) begin their memoir with a well-known riddle joke told by the male soldiers: "What's the difference between a slut and a bitch? A slut will sleep with anyone. A bitch won't sleep with you." This riddle joke captures the dilemma faced by women in the military, where sexual assault is a serious problem. In fact, every account by a female warrior or by a female journalist interviewing female warriors testifies to the constant threat of sexual harassment and assault from male warriors, from sexual assaults by recruiting officers (Thorpe 2014, 65) to assaults by peers and superior officers.

The homoerotic nature of R&T playfighting among male warriors, play that both is and is not fighting and both is and is not sex, serves well the need for the men to bond closely, but such playfighting and its resemblance to sex would not serve the psychological and social needs of the women warriors, sending the wrong message. They need to prove themselves as tough as the men, but they do this by performing well in physical training (Biank 2013, 127) and not by engaging in physical contests with the men.

In conclusion we can say this about R&T playfighting and women warriors. For now, the playfighting is not suited to their bonding needs, and we are unsure whether Gray's distinction between comradeship and friendship among warriors applies to the women. We do know that social and historical forces like the women's movement and concrete changes such as those created by Title IX have made girls' play and young women's play more and more like that of men, that women's sports teams haze members (Mechling 2009), that more and more women are enrolling in ROTC in high school and college, and that the participation of women in sports have made them as physically fit as many men, to say nothing of the socialization that takes place in competitive team sports. As we write these words, the military is close to making new rules for the participation of women members in combat. Women have played combat roles for a few years now, as witnessed in memoirs, reporters' accounts, the documentary film *Lioness* (2008), and Lemmon's (2015) book following members of the all-female Cultural Support Team (CST) in training and on missions with male Special Operations warriors. The full integration of women into combat roles seems very likely, and it will be interesting to watch what happens to the R&T playfighting in those units.

R&T PLAYFIGHTING AND PTSD

We see one other, nontrivial use of R&T playfighting by warriors in combat zones. A large proportion of the warriors returning from service in Iraq and Afghanistan are experiencing symptoms of posttraumatic stress disorder. Called "nostalgia" and "soldier's heart" (American Civil War) in the eighteenth and nineteenth centuries, this syndrome was recognized as "shell shock" in WWI, and as "combat fatigue" in WWII and Korea (Tick 2005, 99). So many Vietnam War veterans came back with the classic symptoms—flashbacks to the traumatic event, emotional numbing, hypervigilance, avoidance of situations resembling the threatening ones, sleep disorders, and irritability (A. Young 1995, 107; Finley 2011, 5)—that the 1980 *Diagnostic and Statistical Manual of Mental Disorders* (the DSM-III) finally named and described posttraumatic stress disorder. As a therapist, Shay (1994, 2002) prefers PTSS (syndrome rather than disorder) and he stresses that the syndrome is symptomatic of a "moral injury" (1994, 20); but he recognizes that we are stuck with PTSD as the acronym.

The entire lay and professional discourse about PTSD in American warriors (including women) arises as veterans experience the symptoms weeks, months, even years later and have to wait for months and years to get the therapeutic help they need. In contrast, our focus here is on R&T playfighting in the combat zone and the possibility that this folk tradition amounts to a sort of immediate or short-term folk therapy. If folklore provides resources for living meaningful lives and for coping with social and psychological anxieties, then we would expect that folk traditions like R&T playfighting (notably in male friendship groups) might at least temporarily ameliorate the combination of guilt, anger, psychic numbing, and depression that follows traumatic events in the combat zone. Folklore can fail, of course.

When warriors return from a dangerous mission or even a routine, stressful day "outside the wire," that is, away from the relative safety of their base, protocol requires that they take care of their equipment first, cleaning weapons and putting away gear. The cleaning of the weapons doubtless has a calming effect in its repetitious movements, movements learned and drilled since basic training. Moreover, the object of concentration and tactile stimulation is the individual's weapon, which (as we have seen) comes to have symbolic importance as a penis, a phallic symbol of power and destruction, rather than creation. In fact, the US military has what amounts to a fetish when it comes to machines in combat, even when the machines seem poorly suited to the nature of the combat setting and requirements.

It is when the "housekeeping" part of the return to base is over that the warriors move on to other post-mission, stress-relieving folk therapies, from the totally solitary one of listening to music on one's iPod to playing video games alone or with others to telling stories and generally "shooting the shit." Therapists who have worked with veterans with PTSD recognize the therapeutic value of telling stories. Even routine, seemingly mundane conversations in the hooch can have the qualities of folklore, of speech and gesture performed for the audience toward a particular end. It is during the boring downtime, with the rush of adrenaline gone or fading, that the playfighting emerges, from the game of gay chicken to the birthday beatdown to blood in, blood out, and to the very physical and rambunctious R&T playfighting recorded in Hetherington's photographs.

We believe that the therapeutic value of these folk approaches in dealing with the trauma and continual stress of the combat zone increases as the folk therapy moves from the highly individual to the very social. A popular therapeutic theory and practice in dealing with PTSD months and years later is a behavioral therapy aimed at reducing the veteran's anxiety through "deconditioning," through a systematic desensitization whereby the therapist helps the veteran return repeatedly to the heightened state of excitement of the traumatic event or extended stress (A. Young 1995, 177), discovering repeatedly that he is not wounded or killed in that heightened state of the flooding of adrenaline, endorphins, and other body and brain-related hormones. Some therapists are even experimenting with elaborate virtual reality reenactments of the traumatic event (e.g., an IED exploding near the warrior's vehicle), taking the veteran through repeated experiences of the sights, sounds, physical experiences, and even smells of the remembered traumatic event, with the veteran narrating the events and his feelings through the simulation (McLay 2012). This PET, though a common approach, is controversial and faulted by therapists—notably those who use psychodynamic therapy to treat PTSD (A. Young 1995, 179)—because PET does not address the contents and meanings of the traumatic memory (Finley 2011, 125).

Cognitive and psychodynamic therapies for PTSD may be quite effective for some veterans in therapy months and (more likely) years later, when it is traumatic memories that must be addressed. But R&T playfighting in the combat zone resembles PET in its re-creation of the physiological and mental states of excitement experienced in combat. The R&T playfighting provides a "safe" frame for experiencing that arousal and for having the experience end with no injuries or death. We are not in a position to know for sure what sorts of therapeutic relief the R&T playfighting brings the warriors, of course, but the warriors engage in this play often enough and enough at risk that we believe they have discovered a folk therapy for reliving and relieving their stress, anxiety, and anger.

CONCLUSION

It is not an accident that Bateson (1972 [1955]) formulated his ideas about frames and about communication and meta-communication while trying to understand playfighting he observed between mammals at the zoo. Playfighting provides a rich example of the paradox of play, and the drive in mammals to playfight seems a further paradox in light of sociobiological theories about the evolution of behavior. The risks of playfighting (including the risk of injury, inattention to external threats, and the expenditure of precious calories) seem to far outweigh the benefits. R&T playfighting among warriors in combat zones seems risky to the point of being what Geertz, borrowing from Jeremy Bentham, calls "deep play," "play in which the stakes are so high that it is, from his [Bentham's] utilitarian standpoint, irrational for men to engage in it at all" (1973, 432). As we have seen, the paradoxical nature of R&T playfighting—that it both is and it not fighting and both is and is not sex—serves the psychological needs and social needs of the warriors. The resemblance between the physiological state of arousal in real violence, sex, and R&T playfighting guarantees that the male warriors will return again and again to the R&T playfighting to help them manage their emotions, including their love for each other on the battlefield.

FIVE
Playing Video Games

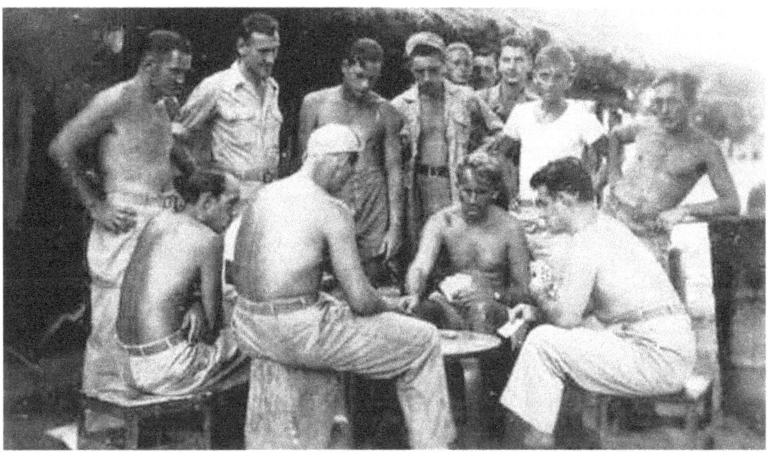

Figure 5.1. Troops playing cards. Mechling collection.

Junger's account in *War* (2010) of the lives of the Marines at Outpost Restrepo, a remote outpost in the Korengal Valley of Eastern Afghanistan, and Hetherington's photographs (collected in *Infidel*, 2010) of that year at Restrepo and the documentary film, *Restrepo* (2010), Junger and Hetherington made of that year embedded with the platoon, document how much those Marines, in a very dangerous outpost, enjoyed playing video games, including *Guitar Hero* and first-person shooter (FPS) games like *Halo*, *Battlefield*, and *Call of Duty*. Many warriors own or share handheld devices (PSPs), and many play multiplayer games on consoles. Playing video games fills the hours distracting the warriors from the endless waiting—waiting for orders, waiting for chow, waiting for contact with the enemy, waiting for sleep, waiting for the end of deployment, waiting, waiting, waiting, endlessly waiting.

Journalist David Finkel was embedded with "the 2–16," Second Batallion, Sixteenth Infantry Regiment, during the "surge" of 2007–2008, when President Bush poured a large number of American troops into Iraq to turn the tide of that war. Here is Finkel's description of the downtime activities of a group of 2–16 soldiers barely a week after they lost a comrade in an IED incident. "A week after Cajimat's death," writes Finkel,

> they were passing time between missions like they usually did, by playing video games on their computers or video-chatting over the Internet. Or lifting weights, or watching bootleg DVDs that they could buy at the hospital for a dollar. Or drinking Red Bulls or Mountain Dews or water mixed with high-protein powder. Or stuffing themselves with tubs of Corn Pops at the dining facility. Or flipping through magazines that came as close as possible to violating the army's ban on pornography. Such was life on the FOB [Forward Operating Base] for the eight hundred of the finest, whose behavior could be explained simply by the fact that so many of them were nineteen, or by the more complicated fact suggested by the ubiquitous blast walls that they did all of these things behind. (2009, 37)

Video games, physical activity like lifting weights, watching movies, consuming as much caffeine and sugar as possible, and consuming porn as fast as the Sugar Pops—not a bad list for us to look for folk therapeutic approaches to stress.

As with the other forms of folk therapy we examine here, video games offer both social psychological benefits and physiological benefits, reducing stress in the warrior. Video games offer some unique elements, though, as we shall see. And video games are such a pervasive phenomenon in American culture that they have become the focus of a great deal of debate about violence in American culture. So we address that debate first before going on to describe the ways the social, psychological, and physiological elements of playing video games serve the warriors' needs beyond entertainment and distraction. We will find in those elements of the games their therapeutic value for giving warriors some relief, however temporary, for the stress of living, working, and fighting in the combat zone.

VIDEO GAMES AND VIOLENCE

Since their evolution from simple games with crude graphics into complex games with extremely realistic graphics, video games have been at the center of fierce public debates about the effects of violent images and song lyrics in American popular culture. The public debate over violent video games is just the most recent chapter in a long history of "moral panics" (as historians call them). Adults worried about the bad influence of "dime novels" on the young men reading them in the 1880s and 1890s, and comic books alarmed parents and teachers and politicians so much in the 1950s that Congress actually held hearings about the menace (B. Wright 2001). Violence in gangsta rap and other musical genres sparked yet another moral panic, and as that debate heated up in the culture wars along came violent video games like *Mortal Kombat* (1992), *Doom* (1993), and *Wolfenstein 3D* (1992). *Grand Theft Auto* (1997) and *Call of Duty* (2003) are just two of the FPS games that agitated adults so much that the industry was forced to put warning labels on the game boxes, just as the music industry was forced to put warning labels—"explicit lyrics"—on the CD cases.

We do not have the space here to rehearse those arguments, but many scholars who have examined the research claiming that violent video games prompt real violence find so many faults with the design and execution of the research that they conclude that there is no evidence of a link between playing the games and becoming aggressive and violent in real life (G. Jones 2002; Markey and Ferguson 2017). The folk idea that popular culture has such a powerful effect on actual audience behavior simply is a folk fallacy.

The moral panics tend to be about children and adolescents (Best 1990), but men and women both play video games well into their twenties, thirties, and some even later. The military recruits men and women precisely from the age group that plays video games, and for that reason the military developed recruiting and training video games to appeal to their potential and actual recruits. Mead (2013) tells this history of the rise of "the military-entertainment complex." The military experimented with game-based training a little before 9/11, but that event led to the creation of a "cutting-edge action video game," a FPS game—*America's Army*—explicitly for recruiting young people (Mead 2013, 74; Allen 2017).

The military's use of video games in training feeds the concern that there is a direct link between the games and actual aggression and violence. There is no such link, but the military games and emerging aspects of actual warfare that resemble the games (notably the use of weaponized drones) fuel the debate.

Not only do we agree with the research that rejects causal links between violent video games and actual interpersonal violence, we argue in this chapter that there are actual positive effects of the FPS and other video games as played by warriors in the combat zone. As we shall see, some psychologists are experimenting with video games as a therapy for veterans suffering moderate-to-severe PTSD, which further suggests to us that the video game play by the warriors in the combat zone serves a therapeutic function for coping with the ore immediate stress.

Let us look first at the social functions of video game play by warriors, especially play in groups.

PLAYING VIDEO GAMES AND MALE BONDING

Playing video games in a group of two or more (dyads can be folk groups [Oring 1984]) serves social bonding needs in the male friendship group, in this case the squad or platoon. Women do play video games, of course, and some women warriors will join in the play. We focus here, though, on the role of playing video games in the male folk group's social construction of their friendships. In the usual gaming situation, two or more players are side-by-side concentrating on the action on the television monitor attached to the game console. Paradoxically, male players experience this side-by-side play as intimate, even though it involves none of the face-to-face eye contact considered necessary for intimate connections in other settings, notably between men and women.

Those who study gender communication (e.g., Tannen 1990) note the ability of American men to experience intimacy doing things side-by-side, whether it is fathers and sons working on a car or other projects or young men sitting on a sofa playing a video game, with all attention on the screen. Wallis experienced this video game bonding both during his two deployments and later, when home, as he and his Marine veteran buddies would gather in his living room to drink some beers and catch up, being sure to include plenty of "trash-talking" during the game play. Wallis reports that his wife was puzzled observing this, as she saw "very little meaningful conversation," and yet Wallis experienced these game sessions as deeply intimate bonding.

As we just noted, a sign of the male-bonding intimacy of side-by-side video game play is the "trash talking" the warriors engage in as players and as spectators. A form of male verbal dueling, "trash talking" involves stylized insults and other playful banter, all understood as communication within the play frame. Whether the game requires cooperation (as in FPS games) or competition (as in *Guitar Hero*), the warriors will "talk trash" to each other throughout the play. The very fact that players can enter into, sustain, and even repair (when necessary) a play frame signals to all involved that they trust each other enough to hurl insults, teases, and taunts that, with a different frame, would amount to "fighting words" (Bateson 1972 [1955]).

FPS games have elements that contribute to their value as a form of folk therapy for traumatic stress in the combat zone. First, when a warrior sits down to play an FPS game, he is guaranteed to make contact with the enemy, something that is distinctly unlike combat. By making contact, we mean that they exchange fire with a hostile force. If every combat unit took contact every day or every time they traveled outside the wire, casualty rates would skyrocket, and military ribbons and medals like the Combat Action Ribbon (CAR), Combat Infantry Badge, and Purple Heart would lose their value. Without a CAR or its equivalent, a warrior is still a "boot" because, according to the Marine Corps, he has not been properly baptized by fire.

In our all-volunteer military, where no one is forced into the infantry, the desire to kill other humans must be present at some point. Casting aside the fact that American warriors are susceptible to the human aversion to kill another human being as discussed by Grossman (2009, 4), video games provide an opportunity to explore the fantasy of killing. For a generation of warriors that grew up with video games and FPS as a part of their adolescence, comparing combat to FPS is inescapable.

Low consequence, a second key feature of the games, offsets the danger inherent in guaranteed contact. While "dying" in a video game is not much of a consequence itself, most game types in FPS involve respawning, allowing players repeatedly to throw themselves back into the battle. Even a highly skilled player with thousands of hours in online multiplayer matches will have a kill-to-death ratio hovering around 2.00 and will have witnessed several thousand deaths of his avatar. This high rate of death and respawning also means that in a standard multiplayer match there will be far more deaths than actual players in the match.

An interesting feature of FPS games is the inclusion of a "Kill Cam" which allows the player to immediately view their own death just prior to being respawned. Depending on the particular game, this kill cam may be from a third-person point of view or the first-person point of view of the enemy that killed them. Players are generally given the option to skip the kill cam in order to respawn more quickly, but a player may use the kill cam to observe the location, weapons, and tactics of the opponent in order to launch a counter offensive. In this way, a death can be actually used to gain a tactical advantage through intelligence gathering, further lowering the overall consequence and detriment of a death.

A third key feature of FPS gameplay is the high level of absurdity of the game. The meaningless and random death and destruction of real combat is compressed and amplified until reaching cartoonish proportions, ensuring a high entertainment factor. This absurdity is a natural result of guaranteed contact, low consequence, and generally endless supplies of weapons and ammunition. While some game types lend themselves to more conservative play by eliminating respawns or lowering the amount of damage a player can take, most matches are fought in a run-and-gun fashion where fast-twitch reactions rule and the intensity of combat remains high for the duration. Games like *Battlefield* (2002) and *Call of Duty* (2003) have generally stuck to contemporary or historical settings and weaponry, so absurdity is achieved through the skill or random luck of players. *Halo* (2001) makes use of a futuristic setting; "Spartan" super soldiers utilizing exoskeletons enable avatars to run faster and jump higher, and cartoonish physics raise further the level of absurdity.

A fourth feature of FPS games is the seamless, error-free operation of any weapon system. Players can focus on just the sensation of release and none of the work that's required to achieve that release. In reality the actual work of employing a weapon system is far more laborious, boring, and difficult. In the first person shooter your avatar is the most technically skilled and flawless weapons operator that ever lived. Not experienced or required are the thousands of hours and rounds required to reach such proficiency with a real weapon system. Gone, too, is the endless cycle of disassembly, cleaning, and reassembly that go into actually putting rounds where you want them.

When exchanging one weapon for another the feel in your hands of the actual manipulation of those weapons is identical; the controller for the video game doesn't change when you pick up a different rifle, pistol, or rocket launcher. In reality, reloading a magazine-fed weapon (not to mention magazines themselves) requires hours of practice. In a video game, if you fire a weapon until the magazine is empty, your avatar completes this action automatically, and any effort on your part can be reduced to pulling the trigger.

Pulling the trigger is the thing a warrior does the least in reality but the most in a video game. In a video game it's all about the release; just spraying bullets everywhere without any thought to conserving ammo, carrying all that ammo, cleaning your weapon, or keeping your weapon in operation by limiting the amount of rounds going through a hot barrel. Additionally, firing thousands of rounds though open-bolt machine guns as a cyclic rate will require that the warrior changes out a hot barrel. This is done to avoid a runaway gun where the barrel gets so hot it literally begins cooking off rounds without pulling the trigger. Warrior game players never see a runaway gun in a video game, let alone an animation where a video game avatar stops shooting to swap out a hot barrel.

It would be disastrous for a video game to have weapons operations be realistic where rounds get stove piped in the chamber or double feeds require that you put a weapon back in action. These added bits of realism might be cool for a second, and some people would appreciate it, but at the end of the day that's not what people want. They don't actually want realism. Gamers would gripe about the algorithm used to determine when a certain weapon had which malfunction, causing endless debate about something that keeps them from what they want to do, which is to pump out rounds.

In a FPS video game, when you get dropped in or spawn into a multiplayer environment or single player for that matter, your player can take far more rounds without dying than any human being. Typically, a player's avatar actually heals over time! There are some hardcore modes where damage in the fight is somewhat more realistic and a single round center mass can put you down, and typically injury is cumulative, but those modes are in the minority.

These features of the games themselves and of the ways warriors in the combat zone interact while playing the games make clear some of the therapeutic benefits of video games. The warriors engage in the male bonding that is so important outside the wire. They can achieve a state of Flow while playing (Csikszentmihalyi 1975). And they can have the odd experience of witnessing their own deaths and resurrections (respawns) over and over again.

Goodman (2013) interviewed Stephen Machuga, founder of the nonprofit Operation Supply Drop (OSD), which raises money to send video games and players to warriors in Afghanistan and Iraq. Machuga, a US Army Ranger with a tour in Iraq, knew firsthand the therapeutic value of playing video games with buddies when back from a mission. Goodman interviewed other veterans who testified to the value of the games provided by OSD. Alan Thomas, a rifle platoon leader, told Goodman (2013),

> I cannot convey the sheer intensity . . . the feeling the understanding between each other that this could be the day where we lose another brother. . . . Even when we get back to camp it's hard to shake that feeling off, even once we ground our boots back on the COP and de-kit. Games did the job to immediately take the edge off. How does one go from a life or death mission to relaxation de-stress time fast enough to have enough mental recuperation for the next round? The OSD [package] I got from Stephen did just that.

Another organization discussed by Goodman (2013), AbleGamers, provides games and game machines to disable veterans, and the effects are the same—helping veterans cope with PTSD and depression.

The Alan Thomas testimony above about the ever-present possibility of death in the combat zone and other comments from veterans suggest that we pause here to consider the complicated ways death plays a paradoxical role in the video games.

DEATH AND REBIRTH

The virtual experience of one's own death and regeneration (resurrection) is a therapeutic experience apart from the resemblance between the arousal and relief experienced in video games and combat stress. This is a huge topic, but an important one for our argument that FPS video game play has short-term therapeutic value for the treatment of PTSD in the combat zone. We make here some succinct, salient points about this psychological phenomenon.

First, the experience of death and rebirth in most of these FPS games resembles the symbolic death and rebirth in most male initiation rituals, and this resemblance is worth noting. Basic training, in most cases, is the warrior's first experience of the death/rebirth motif in male initiations, as the "old" identity is killed and boot camp builds a new identity, a rebirth.

Second, experiencing and reexperiencing one's own death in the FPS game normalizes death for the player; at least that was Wallis's experience. As Grossman (2009) and others note, the key function of basic training is to normalize killing for young people who have a natural resistance to that act. Paradoxically, though, imagining (and watching) one's own death in a FPS game also helps normalize death.

Actually, recruits and warriors will have had a lot of experience watching death in mass-mediated, popular culture television and film. It may be that watching such films also can lead the viewer to imagine his or her own death. Sontag's (1966 [1965]) classic essay, "The Imagination of Disaster," gets at precisely this function of disaster films, the constant experiencing of watching people die, imagining our own deaths, and then not experiencing the real consequences of death. The master of horror fiction, Stephen King, gets at the same truth in his collection of essays, *Danse Macabre* (1980), where King asks why we seek the experience of fright, and his answer is, in part, that the limbic system and the "old," reptilian brain we still bear gets tickled by imagined threat, that horror fiction initiates what we have been writing about in this book—the arousal of the "fight-or-flight" response in our bodies.

The imagination of our own death is a profound experience, one that philosophers, psychologists, and psychiatrists, to say nothing of our greatest writers and artists, have pondered. Elsewhere Mechling (2008b) called this "the Tom Sawyer effect," with reference to the scene in Mark Twain's 1876 novel, *The Adventures of Tom Sawyer*, where Tom and Huck Finn spy on their own funeral from the church rafters. This episode in one of America's most revered novels is powerfully memorable because it reminds us of a secret most of us harbor—the desire to watch the world's reaction to our death.

Ancient philosophers (e.g., the Stoics), and now psychologists, have come around to the conclusion that thinking about death actually has positive outcomes (Beck 2015). This is not to deny the assertions by anthropologists and others that culture in many ways is a human construction meant to create concrete evidence of immortality, to deny the finality of death and its cancellation of meaning. There has emerged, in contrast, a school of thought that thinking about our deaths tames the fear of death and can encourage altruistic action aimed at improving the world. "Terror-management theory" (TMT) emerged as a research field in psychology in the 1980s, and the research on TMT and its therapeutic applications have moved in many directions (Beck 2015; Solomon, Greenberg, and Pyszczynski 2015). The key point for this chapter on FPS video games is that "mindful," conscious thoughts about death help the player be less fearful and, more important, can empower the player (the warrior) to create meaningful relationships in his or her life as a form of immortality—a variant of TMT called the "Meaningful Maintenance Model" (MMM) (Beck 2015). And psychologists who work on a variant of TMT called "anxiety buffer disruption theory" see PTSD as the result of the failure of the human "anxiety buffering mechanisms" (Pyszczynski and Kesebir 2011).

THE BRAIN, BODY, AND VIDEO GAMES

Video games rather easily induce in the player a state of Flow. Csikszentmihalyi (1975) first described Flow as a way to talk about the mental and physical experience of total engrossment in play, the way the play experience induces a state of ecstasy, a stepping aside from ordinary, everyday, taken-for-granted reality and into a reality where time and space take on new dimensions. Csikszentmihalyi is interested in other activities that induce Flow, from rock climbing to brain surgery.

As Csikszentmihalyi conceives it, a player achieves the state of Flow when there is a perfect balance between the difficulty (the challenge) of the activity and the player's ability or skill. If the challenge is great and the ability low, the player experiences anxiety. If the challenge is low in difficulty and the player's skill is high, then the player experiences boredom. Like the surfer (Wallis surfs) who finds the perfect, "sweet" spot in the wave to ride it all the way to the beach, the player catches the wave of Flow and rides the experience, balancing between boredom and anxiety.

Players can set skill levels required for the video game in order to achieve that desired balance between the difficulty of the game challenge and the skills of the players necessary to enter Flow. Video games often provide sets of nested goals that give the player a sense of accomplishment, however small, that entice the player to continue playing.

At its simplest level, then, the engrossment in playing a video game provides escape from the stress. Games do more, though. Holmes and her colleagues (2009) suspected that some "cognitive tasks" can actually interfere with "recently triggered visual memories" of the sort that plague sufferers if PTSD. Having participants in their laboratory experiment play the video game *Tetris*, the authors found support for their hypothesis. Playing the game resulted in fewer flashbacks for a while and may have longer effects. There are many reasons to be cautious about laboratory experiments like this, but given all the recent research on memory it makes sense that tasks taking engrossment, leading to Flow, would occupy certain areas of the brain that would interfere, even briefly, with flashbacks and bad memories.

A relevant body of research on what is happening to the players of video games looks at the chemical and physiological changes in the brain under stress (McLay 2012, 32–37). Traumatic Brain Injuries (TBIs) from nearby explosions, the trauma of witnessing friends' gruesome deaths, the trauma of committing an act of violence, and other traumatic events common in a war zone change the chemistry of the brain and, if prolonged, actually change the physiology of the brain. This is true even without singular traumatic events, as researchers have found that prolonged periods of stress can have the same effects on brain chemistry and physiology.

One psychiatrist working at the Naval Medical Center in San Diego, Robert McLay (2012), sees therapeutic possibilities for treating PTSD in Virtual Reality Exposure Therapy (VRET). Noting the damage to the hippocampus and the amygdala in response to stress, and noting the success some psychiatrists have had treating PTSD with "exposure therapy" and "habituation," McLay describes what is still an experimental therapy, one that draws our attention because its suggests parallels in the folk therapy experiences by warriors as they play video games in the combat zone. Here is one of McLay's colleagues describing his own VRET with Vietnam veterans:

> "It can seem counterintuitive," Dr. Spira conceded. "But we have been using the virtual reality for years to treat Vietnam Vets and other trauma survivors. We teach people to confront the things that they are afraid of. PTSD symptoms build up because you associate real danger with the type of stimuli you just experienced. If you run through the same video sequence enough times without that link to real danger, you realize that the sights and sounds don't hurt you, and it becomes less scary." (McLay 2012, 82)

This prolonged exposure therapy seems to lessen the patient's anxieties and symptoms. Both his conscious and unconscious come to realize that the stimuli that signaled mortal danger in the initial incident did not pose a real threat in his virtual reality reenactments of the incident. We are interested in this work because it helps us understand how playing a video game very soon after the stress of a mission in the combat zone can serve as prolonged exposure folk therapy for the physiological and mental reactions to the stressful mission.

Mead (2013) describes experiments with VRET, and in particular video games designed for therapeutic use with Iraq and Afghan War veterans. He tells the story of Jerry Della Salla, an Iraq War veteran with moderate symptoms of PTSD. Della Salla began working with therapist Michael Kramer at the VA hospital in Manhattan (2013, 131). Kramer included Della Salla along with thirty-four other veterans in a pilot program experimenting with VRET. Now the program extends across the country. Virtual reality programs particular to the terrains and conditions in Iraq and in Afghanistan led to the creation of Virtual Iraq and Virtual Afghanistan simulations (2013, 133). Mead tried the Virtual Iraq simulation and was amazed how realistic the simulations were, including visuals, odors, sounds, even movement (2013, 135). "Throughout a given session," explains Mead (2013, 135), "clinicians are in constant contact with the patient, and they can view what the patient is experiencing on their control screen," monitoring heart rate, galvanic skin response and respiration. Mead then recounts one of Della Salla's sessions and the success of that therapy (2013, 140–42).

Our reason for reviewing this development in the uses of virtual simulations in the treatment of PTSD in veterans should be clear by now. The warriors in the combat zone have discovered on their own that playing video games, especially FPS games that simulate the actual combat actions from which they may have just returned to home base, does much to relieve the stress of living, working, and fighting in the combat zone. The video games they play arouse the same feelings, the same neurological, chemical responses in the body and brain as does the expectation of combat, and, just as in VRET, the warriors have repeated experiences of that arousal and the resulting safety. And as in the VRET, the warriors use the game (we surmise) to learn to monitor and control their fears in arousal.

VIDEO GAMES AND SEX

Early in our work on this book, Wallis emailed to Mechling some thoughts he had on the video games "as a form of masturbatory release for combat stress," connecting two of our chapters (games and masturbation), and it is worth quoting his email at length:

> A young virile man goes to boot camp and somehow does not achieve an erection for 13 weeks. During that time, the Marine Corps does its very best to replace if not confuse his sexuality with the urge to kill. Weapons are sexualized and given female names. Sexual acts become something threatened as violent forms of retribution.
>
> By the time he emerges as a Marine, sex is a mission to be accomplished. Far more important and central to his existence however is the desire, the *need,* to kill. He trains for many months, honing his skills,

> daydreaming about getting sent down range so he can feel the adrenaline rush from hearing incoming rounds and yearning to unleash his pent up sexualized aggression on the enemy. In the barracks he plays first-person shooters, further internalizing and practicing the act of making war.
>
> The Marine and his comrades deploy together and soon he finds that war amounts to a lot of waiting. A whole lot of waiting. And not just sitting idly by, but being on alert for long periods of time, only to return to base not having engaged the enemy. Perhaps he goes to the gym, or spends all night in the MWR [Morale, Welfare, and Recreation center] on the internet, but at some point he is going to seek release from his mental "blue-balls." This may come in many forms but for some it will be in a FPS [first-person shooter game], where finally he can squeeze off as many rounds as his heart desires, delighting in head-shots, throwing in a celebratory and undoubtedly sexual "tea-bagging" of his vanquished enemies.
>
> Or perhaps the Marine and his comrades *did* take contact that day but things didn't go so well. Maybe there are regrets. Maybe they were complacent and bored when the shit hit the fan. Maybe there were issues with distinction and he wasn't able to get a clear shot on the enemy. After returning to base and cleaning weapons and gear he and his comrades jump into a game of *Call of Duty* or *Halo*, where the consequences of a misplaced shot are less significant and the enemies are plentiful, their bodies piling up as controllers vibrating with feedback from weapons firing at the cyclic rate and the artificial but addictive "ding" of head shots satiate at least for the time their lust for carnage and destruction on their own terms.

As Wallis's email suggests, the recruit's and then the warrior's association of the arousal of the threats of combat with sexual arousal begins early and is reinforced in the war zone. In the next chapter we go into detail about how masturbation has some therapeutic value to the extent that sexual arousal resembles the arousal of the fight-or-flight response when on missions in the combat zone. The video games played by the warriors upon their return from missions continues the link between violence and sex.

We see connections between the video games, sexual domination, and pornography. Because a warrior's stash of pornography on the modern battlefield is much easier to transport on a thumb drive or electronic device, a gaming system like the PSP or a device like an iPod touch means that warriors often use the same device to play games that they use for masturbation. The device becomes an electronic substitute or supplement for sexual acts and acts of violence. In one handheld device, the modern warrior can simulate the most intimate of acts between human beings, and in a very short span, experience a glimpse of both the creation and destruction of life.

The warriors playing some video games also can reproduce the real sexualized acts of dominance on the battlefield, such as Marine Snipers treating the bodies of their Taliban enemies to a "golden shower" of urine (Wallis 2012; Mechling 2014). In many FPS games, the player has the ability to change their posture to a crouch, and in some cases the prone position. In games like *Call of Duty* or *Halo*, it is not uncommon to witness a player "tea-bagging" a slain opponent by quickly cycling through stances, simulating the brushing of the dead opponent's face with one's hanging scrotum and testicles (the "tea bag"). And in games where the prone position is an option for one's avatar (onscreen character), players will sometimes simulate sexual penetration of the slain enemy, "corpse humping" in the parlance of the players. That teabagging and corpse humping is not limited to combat soldiers who play FPS games, and that such adolescent displays of sexualized violence are not limited to video games, suggests a strong link between sexuality and violence for not only the warrior in a state of repressed sexuality, but the American male in general.

EROS, THANATOS, AND IMMORTALITY

The sexual play some warriors initiate in the FPS video games invites us to inquire briefly into the connections between violence, sex, and imagining our own deaths. This topic deserves a book-length treatment and, in fact, has received it elsewhere. But here we can raise a few questions and connections (Hedges [2002] devotes an entire chapter to "Eros and Thanatos" in combat).

The topic really is immortality.

Young men (and women, presumably) generally think they are immortal. The scoutmaster of the troop Mechling studied for his book on the Boy Scouts gave the young men (ages eleven to eighteen) his "the three I's" speech when they did something dangerous. "At your age," he would say, "you believe in the three 'I's'—you think you are immune, immortal, and infertile. I don't worry about the last one at Scout camp, but I do worry that you think you are immune and immortal" (Mechling 2001, 93). The military recruits young people and counts on their belief in his or her immortality, a belief that the military has to socialize and discipline, to be sure.

This belief in one's personal immortality faces a serious challenge in the combat zone, amidst so much irrational death. Folklore and culture provide the warrior resources for coping with thoughts of one's own mortality.

Already we have seen one of these folk experiences, the experience of the immortality (continual resurrection) of one's avatar in a FPS game.

SIX

The Jack Shack

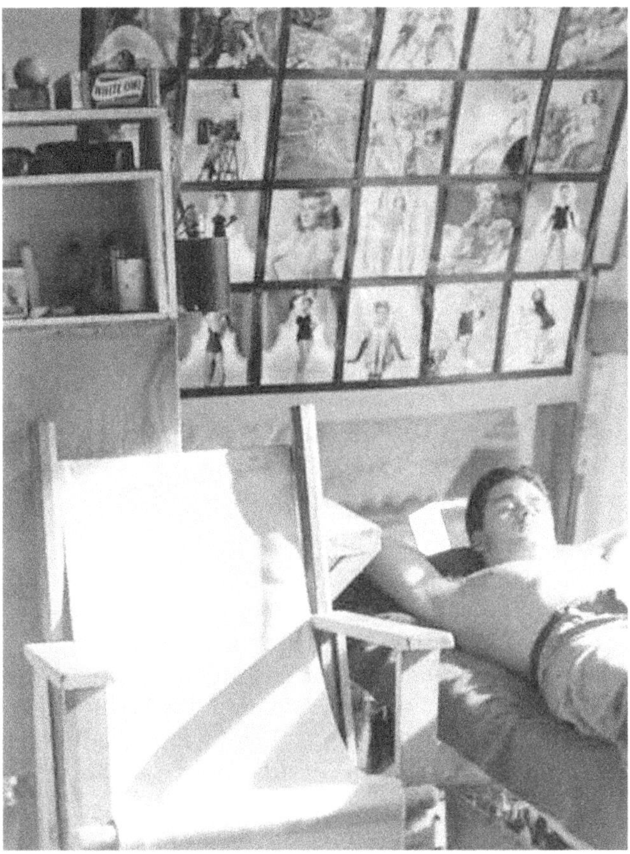

Figure 6.1. Bunk with pinups on wall. Mechling collection.

Men and women masturbate for pleasure, which may be the understatement of this book. They share this behavior with eighty species of primates (including females in fifty of those species), as well as a broad range of other mammals, birds, and reptiles (Kelly 2015). Human males often masturbate from a very young age, discovering the pleasure of touching their penises and getting erections even in infancy. A website maintained by the University of Michigan School of Medicine assures parents that masturbation even at a young age is natural, that many children masturbate by age five or six and by age fifteen, nearly 100 percent of boys and 25 percent of girls have masturbated to orgasm (Viglianco-VanPelt and Boyse 2009). The Michigan website also observes that an estimated 95–99 percent of adult males and 40–60 percent of adult females masturbate. Important for our discussion of masturbation in the military is the fact that men and women masturbate even when sexual acts with other males and females are available.

Medical science confirms what people know from their experiences—namely, that masturbation (like sexual intercourse) arouses a sexual response sequence with four phases: excitement, plateau, orgasm, and resolution. Metaphorically, this sequence of phases resembles the experience of excitement and stress in combat or just on patrols outside the wire, and even if the patrol does not include the "release" of combat and all the hormones that flood the body in the fight-or-flight response, the return safely to base becomes a period of "resolution," a coming down from the tension and excitement.

When a male masturbates, not only are sex hormones and adrenalin involved in the buildup, but the orgasm accompanies "a massive release of the hormone oxytocin from the pituitary gland" (LeVay 1993, 51). The release of oxytocin at orgasm "is under the control of the endorphin system, which is believed to be centrally involved in arousal and pleasure" (LeVay 1993, 52). LeVay also makes the point that the "physiological manifestations and the subjective quality of orgasm seem to be indistinguishable on the two sexes" (1993, 52–53; also Borelli 2014.).

THE FOLKLORE OF MASTURBATION

It may seem odd to include masturbation as a "folk custom" in a book about warriors' uses of folklore to relieve the traumatic stress of living and working and fighting in a combat zone. The key to thinking about masturbation in this way is the physiological resemblance between the state of arousal in sex and the state of arousal in combat or in war zones altogether.

Eating is a natural, biological function meant to address a basic drive (hunger), but sometimes cultures create elaborate foodways—constellations of oral, material, and customary folk traditions—governing eating.

The same is true of the sex drive. Most humans experience that instinctual drive, but the cultural shaping of the sex drive is amazingly varied. It surprises us not at all, then, to find a constellation of oral, material, and customary folklore associated with masturbation. Both men and women masturbate, of course, and cultural histories of masturbation trace the practice and social reactions across a long human history (Laquer 2003; van Driel 2012).

Even without the scholarship, everyone knows that there is a great deal of folklore around masturbation, most of it on male masturbation. Oral folklore includes slang terms (e.g., jacking, jerking, wanking, choking the chicken, spanking the monkey), personal experience stories, jokes (Burns 1984), and contemporary legends (e.g., semen in the mayonnaise at a fastfood restaurant [Langlois 1991]).

Psychologists typically consider young men, ages twelve to twenty-eight, to be "adolescents" in most respects, even though in the United States the age of majority is eighteen. Folklorists see great continuity in the folk cultures of male friendship groups from high school into college (Bronner 1988, 2012), and that college age bracket (ages eighteen to twenty-eight) includes young men in the military, as well. Young men think often about sex, and their sex talk in the male friendship group often includes talk and teasing about masturbation. Whether or not they are actually having sex with women (these all-male total institutions are about the constructions, maintenance, and repair of normative male heterosexuality), men in these groups often will "insult" others as immature males who, unlike the insulter, must resort to masturbation for sexual pleasure. The British term, "wanker," for a male masturbator has entered the American folk speech for the same use—that is, to call another male a "wanker" is a playful insult, suggesting that the target of the insult is less of a man.

In his fieldwork at the annual summer encampment of a troop of Boy Scouts in California, Mechling was serenaded one meeting of the senior scouts (ages fourteen to seventeen) with this parody song (Mechling 2001, 30):

(Tune: "Fanicui, Funicula"—traditional Italian song)
Last night I stayed at home
And masturbated,
It felt so good, I knew it would.
Last night I stayed at home
And masturbated,
It felt so nice, I did it twice.

Chorus

Womp it, stomp it, beat it on the floor,
Wrap it around the bedpost, make it cum some more

Some more, some more, some more, some more,
Some people go for intercourse
But me, I beat my meat! Hey!

Masturbation was on the minds of these young men, at camp in the mountains and far away from girlfriends and other females.

One form of masturbation folklore is bathroom graffiti, a genre first described an analyzed by Alan Dundes (1966). Maximillian Uriarte, in his "Terminal Lance" strip and in his graphic novel about his experiences as a Marine serving in Iraq, notes that the marines he served with drew penises on the walls of their jack shacks, some drawn crudely and some more artfully, most pictured erect and some pictures spurting semen (Uriarte 2016a, 2016b). Dundes's analysis of the motives for graffiti on bathroom walls tends to focus on the symbolism of writing and feces, while Uriarte wonders why Marines are so obsessed with penises.

MASTURBATION IN THE MILITARY

Male warriors serving in Iraq and Afghanistan have appropriated a folk term, "jack shack," for the latrines, portable toilets, and other private places where they can masturbate, often while watching pornographic images on their cell phones, handier sources of visual porn than the "girlie magazines" doubtless used by their fathers and grandfathers for the same reason. The phrase "jack shack" is older slang for a massage parlor or similar establishment where men can pay to be masturbated by a woman, but on US military bases in the combat zone, especially FOBs (forward operating bases), masturbating in the jack shack is a solo adventure. Warriors' memoirs often mention such jack shacks and the men commonly joke with each other about needing the physical release of an orgasm. Rico's (2007) memoir of his tour of duty in Afghanistan recounts how often he and his fellow warriors masturbated in the latrines and showers (50, 90, 97, 180), and he paints a not-so-pretty picture of his sitting in "a shitter" trying to masturbate to the picture of a naked woman on his Palm Pilot, with the smell of feces wafting up from the half barrel under the seat and the sound of other soldiers' pounding on the door urging him to "hurry up" for their own turn masturbating in "the shitter" (2007, 90). Matt Young (2018) devotes as much attention to his and his fellow Marines' masturbation as does Rico. Young even describes and provides illustrations for how the Marines construct a "portable partner" (sometimes called a "portable pussy") out of a towel, a rubber glove, and some rubber bands (2018, 46–52). Young tells of his masturbating while on lookout on a roof at their forward operating base, calling masturbation "a means of survival" (2018, 72).

Obviously, the warriors in Iraq and Afghanistan are not the first soldiers to masturbate in the combat zone. We don't have testimony in memoirs before WWI about masturbation in the combat zone, but one of the most famous memoirs from WWI, Remarque's *All Quiet on the Western Front* (1929), suggests that the German solders and their prisoners of war masturbated regularly. Hirschfeld's book on sex in the Great War, originally published in 1934, describes the "sex hunger" of soldiers in the trenches. Many soldiers relieved the hunger by masturbating (Hirschfeld 1941 [1934], 75–76). He quotes an Austrian soldier who quipped, "Formerly my wife was my right hand, now my right hand is my wife" (77). The author also retells a story about a Bosnian soldier in the Hungarian army who masturbated compulsively in front of his comrades, and Hirschfeld also repeats a report of a French officer who discovered his men masturbating openly while a comrade told a racy story of his wedding night (77).

Hirschfeld (75–76) quotes a long passage from a book by Lissmann (1919) on the effects of war on the sex life of men, including the following:

> During the war a great role was played from the sexo-neurological point of view, by masturbation (ipsalind). In peace times this practice is exceedingly common. It is assumed that ninety-six percent of all young people in the second decade of their life masturbate. But during the war it became far more widespread, according to private and professional records. . . . Indeed, not a few older men who at home were accustomed to regular sexual intercourse, confessed that they had chosen this way of escape from the torture of the senses, to avoid the scruples of conscience, and the dangers consequent upon illegitimate intercourse.

This passage lays out all the reasons why men under stress masturbate in the combat zone—escape from unpleasant senses and memories, escape from the guilt of what they do and see, and avoidance of risky sex with strangers. Nothing has changed in one hundred years.

A query on AskReddit—"Does masturbation occur in the military? Is it non-existent?"—yielded thirty-nine comments by mid-March of 2016, mainly comments from active and veteran military men who testify that, yes, they masturbated in the military, and some offer examples of folklore (Reddit, n.d.). One explained that he and his buddies called it "crying": "Some of us cried in the shower, some of us cried while watching a movie. One guy told me he would use a sock to wipe away his tears. We all cried in the military" (mstevenson53). A submariner (Proud Turtle) reports "jerkoff contests" recorded in notes, and another submariner (pingjockey) notes that there was a chart on the wall beside the weapons launch console keeping track of how many times which crew members masturbated, a story similar to one collected by Raphael (1988, 76) about a "BTMS—Beat the Meat Sheet"—teen boys started at a summer camp to record the number of times each boy in a cabin masturbated. Another comment (ineshidi) offered this motto: "Pooping in a porter john [*sic*] is strong, masturbating in a porter john is army strong." Men in the military often masturbate with socks, and another commentator (rayogata) refers to the "patrol sock." Rico (2007, 100) also mentions a "cum sock" he found in their living quarters.

In both his graphic novel/memoir of his tour in Iraq and his ongoing comic strip, "Terminal Lance," Maximillian Uriarte (2016b) observes the penchant of Marines for drawing penises on the "shitter" (i.e., Porta Potty or other latrine) walls. In one post on his Facebook webpage for "Terminal Lance," (Uriarte 2016a) Uriarte posts a photograph of the door of a Porta Potty from the inside, a brand new portable latrine. His caption for the photo: "Some see a shitter door. Marines see a blank canvas." There follows well over one hundred comments from Marines and other veterans (some active military) about the impulse to draw penises on the latrine walls.

In the comments section responding to a photograph of an army Powerpoint presentation about masturbation, a photo posted on Facebook by "Terminal Lance" author Uriarte, one reader offered this ditty he learned from his father, who flew C-47s in the US Army Air Force in WWII:

> Don't back the attack on the front of a WAC,
> or ride on the crest of a WAVE;
> Just lay on the sand and do it by hand—
> And buy Bonds with the money you save!

While masturbation in the military is usually a solo practice, we do find examples of male warriors masturbating in each other's presence. In one interview by Zeeland for his book, *The Masculine Marine* (1996), the Marine tells of "over the line contests" in which Marines masturbate together to see who "shoots" the farthest when he has his orgasm. When masturbation become a group activity, it serves the homoerotic bonding we discuss at length in our chapter on playfighting.

Finkel (2009) confirms Wallis's observation that the small units had plenty of sexual contraband to enhance the masturbation. Porn on electronic devices and porn in the form of magazines were common, but Finkel also saw an inflatable sex doll and a mail-ordered "pocket pussy" (masturbation sleeve) among the contraband (Finkel 2009, 119, 187). In 2017 a maker of portable masturbation devices marketed the Lifetime Silicone Stroker, "the world's first male sex toy constructed with military-grade materials and designed with the American soldier in mind" (Friederich 2017). Warriors also know how to fashion homemade "pocket pussies" for masturbation, which counts (we suppose) as a folk material culture tradition, but one we would not find in a folklore museum.

The use of sexy "pinup girls" to adorn the living space of warriors has a long history (Gabor 1972). American soldiers returned from WWI with nude postcards widely available in France (Hirschfeld 1941 [1934], 80; Collins 2000; Hoyt 2005, 632), and Goldstein (2001, 334) notes that both

US and British authorities freely distributed to the troops magazine photos of movie stars Rita Hayworth and Betty Grable, defending the practice by saying that the pinup girls "improved morale." Soldiers, airmen, and sailors used the pinup models as sources for the "nose art" they painted on their planes and ships (Ethell and Simonsen 2003). Of course, the "pinup girls" were clothed, sometimes in just a bathing suit, but clothed nonetheless. The military authorities often used images of the popular pinups to convey messages to the troops, including taking care not to reveal secrets to strange women and taking care not to contract a venereal disease (Hoyt 2005). Also popular in WWII were the "Vargas girls," provocative watercolor paintings by Alberto Vargas and appearing in *Esquire* magazine from 1940 to 1946.

The photos in Mechling's collection of vintage snapshots by warriors suggest that the pinup girls by the Vietnam War era were topless, likely taken from the men's magazines, such as *Playboy* (which began in 1953) and *Penthouse* (which began in 1965). In the United States photographs of nude women were not considered pornographic if pubic hair did not show, so until *Playboy* and *Penthouse* broke the barrier and began publishing full-frontal nude pictorials in 1972, most of the pinups of the Vietnam era could be considered soft-core porn. Hard-core pornography was never permitted by the military authorities even in the present wars, which is why the warriors in the Gulf War (1990–1991) and in the wars in Iraq and Afghanistan had to be discreet with their pornography. Wallis (2012) observes that a magazine, *American Curves*, avoided the nudity that would have been banned as pornographic in the Iraq theater of war where he served. That magazine features photographs of athletic and other fit women in bathing suits and other revealing attire. The warriors in Iraq and Afghanistan had to hide their hard-core pornography on their hand-held devices like Palm Pilots, cell phones, and Gameboys, though the enforcement of the rule against possessing pornography varied greatly in time and place. Rico (2007) reports that among the items in the "care packages" people sent to the warriors were *Hustler* and *Penthouse* magazines (along with, we note, a copy of *The Catcher in the Rye*). In 2005, as reported by *Stars and Stripes*, *Maxim* magazine sent twenty thousand copies of the May issue to service members in Iraq (Schonauer 2005).

In earlier wars in other places, American male warriors had access to civilian women for sexual activities (e.g., Roberts 2013), and even before women were as fully integrated into the US armed forces as they now are, male warriors and females in nursing and other support roles could have consensual sexual relations. In some cases in those other wars men could and would have sex with other men, some civilian and some fellow warriors (e.g., Hirshfeld 1941 [1934], 124–40; Cameron 1994, 74–81). And in many of those instances, the men having sex with other men need not necessarily identify themselves as homosexual or even bisexual; men often engage in homosexual acts that they define as situational (e.g., prisons, military), maintaining their identities as heterosexual (Ward 2015).

Sex in the military is a large topic and of current interest because of the public concern about sexual assaults in the armed services, assaults by men against both women and other men. Even setting aside the issue of sexual assaults, the decision to fully integrate women into the military involved debate about the wisdom of introducing the possibility of "fraternization" between the sexes and the possible harm to "unit cohesion" and other issues involved with "the good order and discipline" in the armed services.

The Muslim Middle Eastern societies, particularly where American warriors are doing their duty in Iraq and Afghanistan, levy severe pressure in women to refrain from anything like sexual relations with the American warriors. If a male warrior wants to have consensual sex with a woman or man, that leaves only his fellow warriors, which is against regulations and carries serious punishments. Memoirs and interviews with both male and female warriors who have served tours of duty in Iraq and Afghanistan report that such liaisons do occur, including among sailors at sea, where privacy on a large ship is easier to come by than privacy at a small FOB.

These conditions make all the more important the role of masturbation in the lives of male warriors in the combat zone.

Masturbation violates the military code of conduct. In basic training (boot camp), the recruits are usually too tired to masturbate, even if they could find enough privacy, which is very difficult in the total institution of basic training.

Doubtless, the military has reasons for making masturbation against regulations, as futile as that sounds. It seems that the institution does not enforce the regulation very vigorously, though masturbating while on guard duty (for example) would be a serious breach of rules. We believe that the military's regulations about masturbation stem more from symbolic meanings than from practical reasons having to do with distractions. Laquer's (2003) cultural history of masturbation makes clear the meanings of masturbation after the early eighteenth century, when objections to masturbation changed from moral (Onanism) to ethical and even political (18–19). Masturbation, argues Laquer, was threatening to the ideas of the Enlightenment because masturbation valued secrecy in "a world in which transparency was of a premium" (21), masturbation invites excess, and masturbation has no base in reality because "it was a creature of the imagination" (21).

Those elements and values—imagination, excess, solitude, and privacy—also threaten an institution like the military. From basic training on, the institution suspects privacy and solitude, expects conformity to the reality created by the institution, and expects self-control. What complicates the situation even more for the military is that, as Laquer, explains, beginning

> in the 1970s, solitary sex was regarded as a way of reclaiming the self from the regulatory mechanisms of civil society and of the patriarchal sexual order into which the Enlightenment and its successes had put it. It became a sign of *self*-governance and *self*-control instead of their collapse. (2003, 277)

In terms of generations and generalizations, we might say that the baby boomers (born 1946–1964) grew up in a transitional era and the "sexual revolution" of the 1960s. By the time the genXers (b. 1964–1981) and then the millennials (b. 1982–2000) came along, attitudes toward sex and, in particular, toward masturbation changed considerably, as young people talk comfortably about these matters (e.g., an episode, "The Contest," of television's *Friends* in which the six friends make a bet who can go longest without masturbating).

This progression of comfort with masturbating and talking about masturbating means that the young men entering the military now tend to see masturbation as a healthy expression of the individual self, as a liberation from social controls on sexual behavior and on other forms of individual expression. For these young men, masturbation is not just about the pleasure and release. Masturbation, unconsciously most likely, is about liberation from control, including self-control.

We see this sense of autonomy in some of the humor and stories about masturbation in the military, humor and stories that often feature a soldier's openly defying the military regulations about masturbation. A well-known joke:

> An officer walks in on a recruit who is masturbating in the shower.
> Officer: What are you doing, soldier? Stop that.
> Soldier: Sir, it's part of my body and I can wash it as fast as I want to.

A common military legend is about the soldier who tries to get sent home or otherwise released from the military by seeming to be "crazy" by openly masturbating in front of an officer. In *Full Metal Jacket*, the squad is standing around two bodies of colleagues ready to send off the battlefield, and one's nickname is "hand-job" because of his constant masturbating in front of officers, hoping to be sent home.

In short, while masturbation in the military is a short-term solution to the sexual drives of the young man and may even have some values as a short-term therapy for the stress of living and fighting in the combat zone, masturbation also serves as a prime example of the individual warrior's using his own body to resist the control and uniformity of a total institution.

MASTURBATION AND POSTTRAUMATIC STRESS

Sexaholism—compulsive sexual behavior—is a common symptom in the cluster of behaviors therapists find in veterans, as veterans suffering from PTSD strive to numb their pain with alcohol, other drugs, risky behavior, and sex, all meant to take the veteran into a transcendent state (Tick 2005, 123). Reasoning backward from this symptom of PTSD, we concluded that warriors would seek sexual excitement and release—the transcendent state—in the combat zone as a folk therapeutic solution to the stress.

The French famously call the sexual orgasm "la petite mort," "the little death." That phrase recognizes the state of ecstasy experienced during orgasm and recognizes, as well, the resemblances between the experience of the body during sex or masturbation and the experience of the body in stressful and traumatic situations, like combat,

We include masturbation as form of immediate folk therapy for the stress of living and fighting in a combat zone because, like other genres of play we discuss in this volume, the physiology of arousal and orgasm resembles the physiology and even release experienced in combat. Our premise here is that the bodily sensations experienced in masturbation strongly resemble the sensations aroused in PET for PTSD. This claim rests on the resemblance of arousal in combat and arousal in sex.

In memoirs, novels, and other testimony, veterans often liken the experience of combat with the experience of sex. Many memoirists, journalists, and therapists admit the erotic nature of combat (Tick 2005, 20). In a chapter entitled "Killing at Sexual Range: 'The Primal Aggression, the Release, and the Orgasmic Discharge,'" Grossman uses interviews with veterans to show how sex and death are close kin (2009, 134). "One American soldier compared the killings at My Lai to the closely linked guilt and satisfaction that accompany masturbation" (136), and Grossman quotes another American soldier as saying that "To some people carrying a gun was like having a permanent hard-on. It was a pure sexual trip every time you got to pull the trigger" (2011, 136). Grossman found soldiers quite explicit in comparing "the power and pleasure of explosively spewing a stream of bullets . . . to the emotions felt when explosively spewing a stream of semen" (2009, 136).

This level of conscious observation on the similarity of male sexual experience and the experience of combat taps the actual physiological responses of the body as it is aroused in sexual experiences or in combat. We discussed that physiology earlier, but it helps to review here that hormonal cascade under stress to make our point about sexual arousal as a form of PET.

Scientists have studied the physiology of the male body in combat for many years. The phrase "fight-or-flight" was coined by Harvard physiologist Walter Bradford Cannon (1871–1945) in his 1915 book, *Bodily Changes in Pain, Hunger, Fear, and Rage: An Account of Recent Researches into the Function of Emotional Excitement*. Other medical scientists have built on this work to give us a full understanding of the chemical and accompanying psychological reactions when a mammal faces a serious threat, such as combat (Sapolsky 2004, 19–36). The sympathetic nervous system in human and nonhuman animals begins secreting various hormones from the adrenal medulla (the core of the adrenal gland), including a family of catecholamines that include norepinephrine and epinephrine (other terms for adrenaline and noradrenaline), which function to "mobilize" the brain and body for action. As Sapolsky (2004, 22) puts it, the sympathetic nervous system "helps mediate vigilance, arousal, activation, and motivation." Other hormones elicited in the "fight or flight" response include estrogen, testosterone, cortisol, dopamine, and serotonin. Sapolsky (2004, 30–32) emphasizes the role of glucocorticoids (steroid hormones) in responses to stress. With the experience of stress or even the anticipation of a stressful situation, a chain reaction moves from hypothalamus to the pituitary gland to the adrenal gland, each gland along the way secreting a hormone that signals the next glad to secret its chemicals. And important for the parallel with sexual arousal, the pituitary and brain "also secrete a class of endogenous morphine-like substances called *endorphins* and *enkephalins*, which help blunt pain perception among other things (Sapolsky 2004, 32).

In this age of sophisticated brain imaging and brain science, we know that the physiology of arousal in stress brought on by living in the combat zone and the physiology of sex are remarkably similar. The stage of sexual arousal (toward orgasm) releases neurochemicals that flood the body and brain (the amygdala, the cerebellum, and the pituitary gland, in particular) with feelings of euphoria (Borelli 2014). The relevant hormones resulting in euphoria in the male are testosterone, oestradiol, and certain peptides (ocytocin (OT), beta-endorphons, and prolactin) (Bancroft 2005). Testosterone also plays an important role in the "fight-or-flight" arousal in male warriors who are facing threats. In that aroused state the adrenal medulla produces norepinephrine and epinephrine.

WOMEN, MASTURBATION, AND PTSD

Women masturbate for pleasure too, and although we have plentiful testimony from male warriors and veterans about the ways masturbation serves at least temporarily as a transcendent escape from the stress of living, working, and fighting in the combat zone, we have precious little direct evidence from women warriors and veterans that they also resorted to masturbation as short-term PET-like therapy for stress. None of the war memoirs by female veterans mentions masturbation, and we can speculate why.

Women had a lot of cultural history to overcome in order to be comfortable masturbating and talking about masturbating. The women's movement of the 1960s made the sexual liberation of women a key feminist goal. Through books like *Our Bodies, Ourselves* (Boston Women's Health Book Collective 1973) and Betty Dodson's books (1974, 1987) and workshops for women, feminist activists and writers worked to reverse the patriarchal view of the woman's body and of what sort of sexual activity was appropriate for women. In the 1960s climate of sexual liberation, women were to take their sexual pleasure into their own hands (so to speak) and to claim a right to sexual pleasure, including orgasms. Celebrating masturbation by women and, in some cases, teaching women how to masturbate (e.g., Dodson's workshops) were important in women's wresting control of their own bodies from men.

Many women in the military for the past one hundred years doubtless masturbated for the same reasons Lissman found among the male soldiers in the First World War. Though they did not take combat roles in that war, women served as nurses and other support roles that would have subjected them to the sorts of stress that brings on PTSD, and because the endocrinological events of masturbation in women is the same as in men, we assume that women could find stress relief in masturbation. The advantage those women had (and still have in a total institution like the military) over men is that women can masturbate much more clandestinely. Still, studies show repeatedly that women masturbate less than men (Mintz 2011).

The sexual liberation of women in the 1960s and 1970s meant that women serving in the Vietnam War may have felt more comfortable with masturbation than did their mothers and grandmothers. Certainly by the Gulf War (1990–1991), a war in which women began playing roles in combat as well as support roles, the late baby boomer (born 1946–1964) and early genX women (born after 1964) would have been raised in a culture where the rights of women, including the right to control their sexuality and pleasure, would have been taken for granted. This would be even truer for the women in the wars in Afghanistan (2001–present) and Iraq (2003–present).

Without any evidence provided by women warriors and veterans, we are left to speculate that masturbation can be as useful a short-term therapy for stress in women in the combat zone as for men. Stress-response hormones "are not gendered" (Goldstein 2001, 157), and although there are slight differences in the endocrinology of sexual arousal in men and women (Bancroft 2005), their orgasms are similar (Fogel 2010). Most (maybe all) of the research on sex addiction (sexaholism) in war veterans with PTSD speaks to the male veterans, even though the researchers acknowledge that women experience the symptoms of PTSD in greater numbers than do the men. We need more research on the similarities and differences in the sexual addiction of male and female veterans suffering from PTSD.

CONCLUSION

Yes, we just wrote an entire chapter on masturbation as a folk tradition in the military, a folk tradition that has short-term therapeutic value because of the similarity between the bodily arousal and release in sex and the bodily arousal and release in combat.

SEVEN

Dark Play and Deep Play

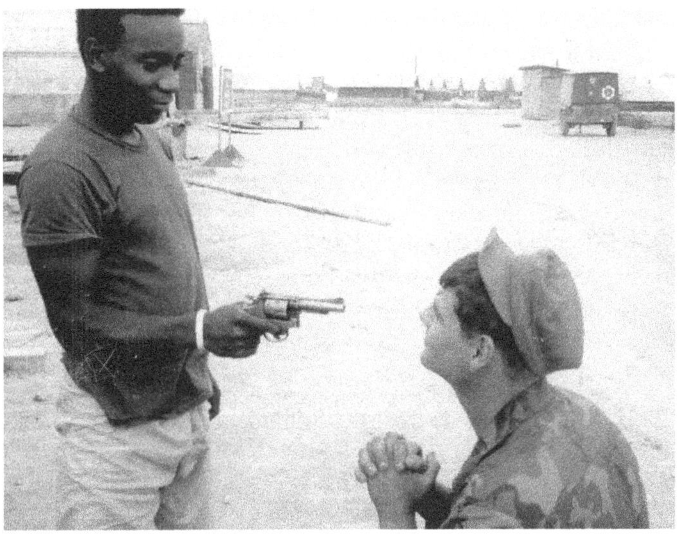

Figure 7.1. Kill the beast. Mechling collection.

In previous chapters we have explored the uses of folklore as a folk therapy for warriors' dealing with the anxieties and symptoms associated with PTSD. The folk traditions covered in those chapters—including the use of pet animals, playfighting, video game play, and masturbation—are all relatively benign compared with the folk traditions we examine in this chapter of "dark play" and "deep play." We feel obliged to warn the reader that the human behavior we describe and analyze in this chapter often is disturbing, sometimes mildly disturbing but at other times horrifying. The reader actually can skip this chapter and still understand the main thesis of this book. But the folklore and folk behavior we examine here is a real part of the lives of warriors, and we owe it to those warriors to listen to what they say and think about what they do to cope with emotions raised in battle. We authors feel a moral imperative to tell this part of the warriors' and veterans' story, to peer into the darkness of battle and the darkness of human nature to understand as fully as we can what it means to be a warrior.

Because so much of what we have to say in this chapter implicates the human body, the warrior's body, we begin with an introduction to how anthropologists, sociolinguists, and folklorists talk about the human body as a symbol of society, and that leads us to some special observations about the warrior's body and the psychological meanings of the wounded body. We then move on to examine "dark play" and "deep play," distinct forms of play in some ways but also overlapping categories. Thus, while gallows humor does not carry great risk to the warrior and is simply "dark play," true "deep play" involves considerable risk to the player.

We begin with the body.

THE TWO BODIES

The anthropologist Mary Douglas (1966) establishes most clearly our understanding of the human body as a symbol of society. There are, as Douglas would say, "two bodies" when we look at the military. There is the individual warrior's body—we focus here on the male body—and there is the "corps," the collective "body" that is the military unit. Douglas explains that the human body is a "bounded" system, with an inside and an outside. The boundary is the skin, with a few openings. For the body, anything that crosses the boundary between outside/inside poses a danger, possible "pollution," and cultures create taboos and rituals for dealing with those dangerous substances and the dangerous moments of transition, when the materials are suspended "betwixt and between" (as Turner [1967] says) one state and another. Thus, cultures create taboos and rituals around things that cross into the body, such as food and drink, and taboos and rituals around things that leave the body, including urine, feces, semen, menstrual blood, blood, milk, tears, sweat, and saliva. Cultures vary on which substances they consider dangerous and how severe are the taboos, but the power of the body as a symbol of society is clear. Like bodies, societies have boundaries and protect the inside from "pollution" from the outside. Clean and dirty are key categories for both bodies and societies. Lakoff and Johnson (1980) show how many of the metaphors we use every day are based in the body, and Sontag's books *Illness as Metaphor* (1978) and *AIDS and Its Metaphors* (1989) show how the metaphors from each realm—the ill body and the ill society—bleed into each other.

The male body is both real flesh and a symbol. Bordo (1999) uses the example of the penis to make an important point about the relationship between the real and symbolic when it comes to male bodies. The penis is a biological organ, but the penis is also a cultural construction (Meching 2008a). The penis "has a symbolic 'double' that is entirely the creation of the cultural imagination: the phallus" (Bordo 1999, 84). Bordo reviews briefly the history of the phallus as a symbol of male strength in Western culture, beginning with the Osiris myth in ancient Egypt and continued by the Greeks in their Dionysian rituals and symbols (1999, 87). Anthropologists offer many examples of the symbolic phallus in other cultures beyond the West. Everywhere the phallus is a symbol of strength.

Important for our argument is how the phallus permeates the discourse of males, from talk in their small friendship groups to phallic images in advertising, to phallic images in nationalistic (especially war) propaganda. Christina Jarvis (2010, 44–55) analyzes and illustrates the use of the hard, muscular male body in American propaganda leading up to and during WWII. In the visual embodiments of that "rhetoric of muscles," the bodies of the men and the machines of warfare are fused, such that the large guns and the large shells the soldiers are loading into the guns become the American phallus for the hard bodies.

From their youth boys develop metaphors and other ways to talk about their bodies and those metaphors always portray the body as "hard," as machine-like (Murphy 2001), Boys watch mass-mediated narratives and images featuring strong, "hard" bodies in television, film, and video games. By the time young men are adults, they understand fully that the American cultural ideal is for them to have strong, hard bodies. Just as cultural ideals about what the female body should look like sometimes results in eating disorders in young women, so the cultural ideals about the male body often create the young man's dissatisfaction with his body, his feeling that his body does not have enough bulk, strength, is not "hard" enough. And any stroll through a fitness club demonstrates the striving for a harder body in men, the "muscle dysmorphia" that drives the quest for more muscles, harder muscles, and (hence) more masculinity (Bordo 1999, 221).

One "problem" for men is that they have real penises, and one form of the dissatisfaction men feel with their bodies is that their penises are not large enough. "The phallus," writes Bordo (1999, 95), "haunts the penis. Paradoxically, at the same time the penis—capable of being soft as well as hard, helpless as well as proud, emotionally needy as well as a masterful sexual performer—also haunts the phallic authority, threatens its undoing."

Bordo's book and others (e.g., Jeffords [1993], on "hard bodies" in the films of the Reagan years) document the narrative and visual environment in which American boys grow up and then live their lives as adult men. Which brings us back to the socialization of young males (chapter 1) and the centrality of the male body in their construction of their masculinity.

By the time the young male enters the military, he understands fully well the cultural ideal of the strong, hard body. Basic training (boot camp) only intensifies the recruit's fixation on his body. The military is a "total institution" (Goffman 1961), and boot camp is the most closely controlled setting in the military, with total control over the recruit's body. The institution shaves his head and takes complete control over his bodily functions, from eating and sleeping to urinating and defecating. Physical training (PT) in boot camp is all about creating a strong, hard, warrior's body. In fact, the recruit's thinking about his own body melds with his thinking about the weapon he is issued, personifying the weapon and taking as much care in keeping it clean and in working order as he does his body. The male recruit has a penis, but his weapon is a phallus.

THE WOUNDED BODY

Having established the symbolic power of the male body, especially the male warrior's body, we need to make one more important point in preparation for our discussion of dark play and, especially, deep play. One thing male warriors know for sure is the fragility of the male body. This was "Snowden's Secret" in one of the most powerful episodes in Heller's *Catch-22* (1961), his novel/memoir of being a bomber pilot during WWII over Italy. Late in the novel Yossarian, the central character and pilot, crawls back in the bomber to attend to the wounded gunner, Snowden. Yossarian calmly treats Snowden's thigh wound from shrapnel, thinking he has saved Snowden, when he (Yossarian) suddenly realizes that there is a far more serious wound under Snowden's flak suit:

> Yossarian ripped open the snaps of Snowden's flak suit and heard himself scream wildly as Snowden's insides slithered down to the floor in a soggy pile and just kept dripping out. . . . Yossarian . . . gazed down despondently at the grim secret Snowden had spilled all over the

> messy floor. It was easy to read the message in his entrails. Man was matter, that was Snowden's secret. Drop him out a window and he'll fall. Set fire to him and he'll burn. Bury him and he'll rot, like other kinds of garbage. The spirit gone, man is garbage. That was Snowden's secret. Ripeness was all (Heller 1961, 439–40).

The war memoirists sometimes comment on "Snowden's Secret," not calling it that, but observing in the carnage they witness the fragility of the human body.

We have seen in earlier chapters that a central, powerful element of being a warrior is a valorization of pain. Suffering and sacrifice, claims O'Connell (2012, 29), are reframed as pleasure in the Marine Corps; the drill instructors regularly define pain as "fear leaving the body." Once in the combat zone, fear for one's body becomes paramount. Jarvis's (2010) book on the male body in WWII devotes an entire chapter to "Representing Wounded Bodies," including what the warriors think about wounded bodies. War memoirs up to the present are filled with descriptions of wounded bodies, mangled and torn-apart bodies of both enemies and friends. Many observers mention the pornographic nature of this fascination with "war porn."

Given the salience of the male body at war and anxiety about the body, it should not surprise us that bodies figure prominently in the folk practices of black humor and "deep play," which we explain shortly. First we turn to humor.

BLACK HUMOR AND GALLOWS HUMOR

Folklore in its various forms—oral, material, and customary—helps people deal with the social and psychological anxieties that come up in everyday life. And many of these anxieties arise in the close, high-context folk groups that we move in and through in our everyday lives. Families, friendship groups, and workplaces are primary sites for the working of folklore to keep those groups bonded, and humor is a common folk resource for dealing with social and psychological stresses in those folk groups. Humor in the folk group—that is, humor as it is actually employed in a live performance in a group—is a form of play, and as we saw in the chapter on playfighting, a great advantage of the play frame is its subjunctive mood, it's "what if?" quality where things do not mean in the play frame what they would mean in another frame, such as everyday life.

As a form of play, humor has the same advantages. People employ humor in the high context folk group to accomplish many things in managing the relationships between the people in the group. Humor in a folk group has value in being impersonal, indirect. If a member of the group wants to comment on another member's behavior, for example, but if that comment would create strife within the group and threaten its cohesion, humor can be an indirect way to make the comment. Humor and jokes sometimes fail, in which case the person performing the humor can always say, "It's just a joke."

The members of the military folk group, the friendship group of the team or squad or platoon, routinely use humor to manage their interpersonal relationships. Scholars refer to the "license to joke" (Mechling and Mechling 1985) as a way of acknowledging that the teller of a joke and the audience enter into a joking frame (a play frame) in which it is understood that the jokes are not to be taken seriously; they are told in fun. And the humor does not have to be in the form of a formal joke; there are other genres of humor we would find in the military folk group. As in the play frame, the very fact that people enter into a joke frame signals to them that they have a close, trusting relationship. Like any play frame, the joking frame is somewhat fragile and can be broken easily. If the participants (teller and audience) wish to maintain their relationships, they will repair the communication event in the event the joke offends or otherwise fails.

Folklorists and other scholars of humor have been studying gallows humor for a long time (Obrdlik 1942). Freud (1961 [1927]) recognized that an important function of humor is as a defense mechanism in the face of anxiety, stress, and trauma. Oppressed groups often resort to gallows humor, and people can joke in some of the most awful circumstances, such as prisons, concentration camps, wars, and natural disasters (Jackson 1965; Lipman 1991).

Warriors use "black humor," sometimes called "gallows humor," as a way of coping with the extreme stress of the combat zone. Black humor responds to the absurdity of war, to the irrationality of life and death. The common phrase, "there it is," used by warriors in Vietnam to comment on some event (usually an irrational death) summarizes in a pithy phrase the irony in the event. Another common phrase used by Vietnam warriors and veterans is "It don't mean nothin,'" a different way of acknowledging the absurdity and meaninglessness of the war they are fighting (Shay 1994, 38; Finkel 2009, 93; Tick 2005, 93). Kurt Vonnegut's narrator in *Slaugterhouse-Five* (1969), his novel of WWII based in part on his own POW experience in Dresden during the horrific firebombing of that city, utters the phrase "so it goes" repeatedly throughout the novel, achieving the same economical observation as "there it is."

Black humor comes in longer, more elaborate forms, though. Finkel (2009) gives us a few examples from his time embedded with the 2–16. He saw some warrior had fashioned a handmade "morale meter with seven settings," including "Embracing the suck," "Fuck this shit, I quit," and "Bend over. Here it comes again" (90). He witnessed the warriors in a Humvee on a mission playing a game of "last words." What did the men want their last words to be? "Kill 'em all." "Fuck Nine-eleven." "Tell my wife I really didn't love her" (121). The warriors Finkel lived beside called any body found in the water "Bob," for "bobbing in the float," usually a sewage ditch (48).

Joseph Ward (1991, 19–20) and his fellow recruits in basic training at Camp Pendleton witnessed another recruit's suicide-by-M-14 on the firing range. The platoon's drill instructor immediately called over Ward's group and instructed them on the proper way to commit suicide, standing under a cold shower and cutting their forearms from wrist to elbow, holding them high above their heads. "Neat and clean, do you understand?" They did. Certain "playful" acts have the elements of black humor, as when the Marines in Wallis units played on the Marine mantra in the desert, "hydrate or die," by placing water bottles in the hands of dead insurgents.

The only reasonable response to the absurdity of war is to tell and retell stories about the absurdity. The stories veterans tell their therapists often were told first to colleagues in downtime at base camp. Shay (1994, 138) and Tick (2005, 113) heard and retell many of these stories.

Sometimes we find the black humor in the tattoos on warriors' bodies. The documentary film, *Tattooed Under Fire* (dir. Nancy Schiesari, 2009), is set in a tattoo parlor in Killeen, Texas, the home of the army's Fort Hood, and the film features male and female soldiers headed to the combat zones in Iraq and Afghanistan and those recently returned home from those theaters of war. The film provides dramatic examples of this black humor on skin. Travis, a medic we see both before his deployment and upon his return home, requested a unique, disturbing tattoo on his upper arm—a fetus in a blender. Travis understood that the tattoo was offensive, especially to fellow soldiers who have children, but he defended the tattoo as expressing precisely how he envisioned his coming experience in Iraq, as an innocent, helpless fetus being chopped up in a blender. Another soldier interviewed in that same tattoo parlor showed and talked about his tattoo of a baby "grim reaper" with a pacifier in its mouth, carrying a reaper's scythe. That soldier had killed a child in Iraq and the memory haunts him.

Black humor, while it may disturb some, is benign in its motives. Deep play is more complicated and more risky.

DEEP PLAY WITH WEAPONS

Anthropologist Clifford Geertz, borrowing from Jeremy Bentham, writes about Balinese cockfighting as "deep play," "play in which the stakes are so high that it is, from his [Bentham's] utilitarian standpoint, irrational for men to engage in it at all" (1973, 432). One form of deep play is dangerous play. Warriors' memories and reminiscences are full of examples of dangerous deep play, play that reproduces the physiological and mental arousal experienced in combat. Deep play, risky play, can trigger the adrenaline rush experienced in combat (Finley 2011, 58). Risky play can induce a state of Flow (Csikzsentmihalyi 1975), a state of such engrossment that the player loses all sense of time and space, that the player experiences ecstasy (*ex stasis*), stepping away from ordinary reality.

Mechling's collection of vernacular photography (snapshots) by warriors includes several examples of deep play with weapons, a visual record extending back to WWI. Sometimes the weapons are bayonets fixed on rifles. In numerous snapshots one or more warriors are pointing handguns and rifles at others. The likelihood of actual harm in these posed vignettes involving weapons is slim, but it is always a possibility. Mechling's brother-in-law was actually shot in the face (he survived) when he and some army buddies were playing with a handgun in a barracks in Germany, and it will surprise nobody that alcohol adds to the risky, hence deep, play.

DEEP PLAY—SELF-HARM

Death by risky deep play may be a form of suicide among warriors and veterans. After participating in a disturbing atrocity with his platoon—a firefight in which they mistakenly slaughtered many women and children—Vietnam memoirist Kovic (1976) thought about another Marine who stepped on a booby trap and was wounded enough to be sent home. So he, Kovic,

> started to look for booby traps to step on, taking all sorts of crazy chances, trying to forget about the rain and the cold and the dead children and the corporal. I would go off alone sometimes on patrol looking for traps, hoping I'd get blown up enough to be sent home, but not enough to get killed. It was a rough kind of game to play. I remember walking along, knowing goddamn well exactly what I was doing, just waiting for those metal splinters to go bursting up into my testicles, sending me home a wounded hero. (1976, 204)

War memoirs and novels and other testimony are full of stories of warriors' harming themselves in hopes that their wounds will be a ticket home (Dokoupil 2008). Self-mutiliation in the combat zone is risky business. Aside from the risk of harming oneself too much, self-mutilation was a summary execution offense in WWI and still is in some military organizations.

Rotunda and Freilich (2014) review current US military regulations and argue that the Uniform Code of Military Conduct unfairly and unwisely punishes warriors who commit self-injury or who actually attempt suicide. We shall discuss attempted suicide below, but more immediately we want to consider whether and how self-injury amounts to a kind of folk therapy for PTSD.

Non-suicidal self-injury violates two articles of the Uniform Code of Military Justice (UCMJ). "Article 115," explain Rotunda and Freilich (2014, 427), "criminalizes 'malingering,' which includes 'intentional infliction of self-injury for the purpose of avoiding work, duty, or service.'" "Article 134," they continue, "called 'the general article,' is an extraordinarily broad and unusual catch-all, criminalizing 'all disorders and neglects to the prejudice of good order and discipline in the Armed Forces' and 'all conduct of a nature to bring discredit upon the Armed Forces.'" Warriors' memoirs and novels record examples of the sort of self-harm the UCMJ would hold as conduct punishable by Court-Martial. In Goolsby's (2015, 135) novel about young men who go to war in Afghanistan from Northern California, for example, one of the characters stabs himself in the foot and cuts off toes in order to be sent home. Near the end of the ultimate combat scene in Oliver Stone's theatrical Vietnam War film, *Platoon* (1986), one of the characters intentionally stabs himself in the thigh with a knife to be able to have a non-lethal wound that would send him safely home. And Rieckhoff (2006, 129) recounts working to save a soldier under his command, a soldier who shot himself in the leg with an Iraqi pistol in hope that the "million dollar" nonlethal wound (as warriors call such wounds) would be his ticket home.

This discussion, moving toward a consideration of self-injury as a form of folk therapy for combat stress, requires us to make the case that self-injury, self-mutilation, can be considered a folk practice. This is a complicated question.

Sociologists Adler and Adler (2011) interviewed dozens of people who engage in self-injury (SI, also called self-harm in Europe) in order to understand the phenomenon. Most of their informants engaged in cutting, branding, and burning, with a few practicing scratching, bone-breaking, bruising, and picking. Whereas SI, especially cutting, for years was considered by mental health experts to be a "borderline personality disorder" (DSM-5, 2013), a symptom connected to a range of disorders, including PTSD, broad publicity about SI in the 1990s began a reconsideration of SI. Now mental health professionals and others see most cases of SI as a "coping strategy" employed by "capable" and "resilient" people who have suffered trauma, usually in their childhood or youth, and who find relief in the SI (Adler and Adler 2011, 25). The Adlers see SI as a form of "self-help," in the terms we would use here, as a form of self-therapy to review the symptoms of stress and trauma. "Self-injury," write the Adlers,

> tends to lead to the lessening of tension, cessation of depersonalization (grounding), euphoria, improved sexual feelings, diminution of anger, satisfaction of self-punishment urges, security, uniqueness, manipulation of others, and relief from feelings of depression, loneliness, loss, and alienation. It provides a sense of control, reconfirms the presence of one's body, dulls feelings, and converts unbearable emotional pain

> into manageable physical pain. As such, it represents an emotion-regulation strategy (Adler and Adler 2011, 25).

Cutters often report feeling something like the dissociation from the body we find in other ecstatic states, something like the experience of a state of Flow (Csikszentmihalyi 1975) we find in other activities.

Women who engage in SI tend to "turn pain and hostility inward, while men externalize their hurt and engage in outwardly destructive behavior" (Adler and Adler 2011, 24). As we saw in the earlier chapter on the socialization of boys, anger is one of the few emotions adults permit boys to express, so the pain and anger experienced in SI by young men satisfies the need to express those emotions (Adler and Adler 2011, 13, 24). Of special interest for our purposes here is the observation by the Adlers that SI can be an important element in male bonding. "Particularly common in athletic or other hypermasculine subcultures," they write, "young men engaged in various injurious acts, probably the most common being self-burning, to prove that they were tough and could take the pain. This reinforced their identity and connection to the group" (Adler and Adler 2011, 13). "Group branding rituals," common in male friendship groups, especially African American fraternities, seal the male's bonding to the group in pain.

Cutters and branders usually are ashamed of their behavior and mark their skin with scars in places easily covered by clothing. Self-harm in the form of cutting and branding has become an issue for the US Military because some men and women wishing to enlist still bear the scars from self-harm in their younger years. This dilemma resembles the evolving attitudes in the military toward tattoos. At present, the official position of the armed services is that they will not waiver recruitment standards to accept applicants with a history of self-mutilation (Dickstein 2017), though we have some anecdotal evidence that in individual cases the military will require men and women who wish to enlist but who have visible scars from SI to undergo psychological testing to certify their fitness for service (see M. Myers 2018).

Time and again in veterans' memoirs and other testimony, we see the role of pain in the construction of the warrior, especially the male warrior. "Pain is just fear leaving the body," countless drill instructors tell their fresh recruits in basic training, and when Marine veterans gather to tell stories, those stories often feature the pain experienced together and the bonding brought about by the shared painful experiences (Wallis and Mechling 2015). Paradoxically, the male warrior experiences pleasure in the pain.

Although branding is against military regulations, we know it still takes place among male warriors. Swofford (2003, 50–51) was the victim of a prank played on him in basic training when friends pretended they were going to brand him with a hot wire coat hanger, and in Wallis's mortar platoon in Iraq his fellow Marines often gave themselves brands resembling Ruffles potato chips, searing their flesh on the cooling fins that ring the hot mortar tube, a visible sign of belonging to the fraternity of that platoon.

It seems, then, that the more severe forms of self-harm by warriors in the combat zone, acts meant to help the warrior escape from the danger of combat and be sent home, really lie on a spectrum that includes tattooing, branding, and other forms of body modification increasingly common in the younger generations being recruited for the military. Self-inflicted pain amounts to a folk therapy in the combat zone, a form of self-help that brings relief, temporary as it might be, from the anxiety, anger, depression, loneliness, and grief over the loss of friends that is part of daily life in the combat zone. Evidence of SI among warriors in the combat zone is scant, for obvious reasons, but it doubtless occurs as a variety of risky "deep play." Military physicians, note Rotunda and Freilich (2014, 422–23), "have also documented a rising trend in non-suicidal self-injuries, like habitual self-cutting, attributed to 'long, repeated combat tour' and 'strong feelings of desperation.'"

Given the role of SI in emotion management, as the Adlers discovered, it would surprise us if SI is not common in the combat zone. If the evidence of SI among male warriors in the combat zone is scant, the evidence for women warriors seems to be nonexistent.

Most of the self-harm done by warriors in the combat zone is non-suicidal, a somewhat rational act meant to take the person out of harm's way. But Kovic's account of wandering through a minefield hoping to injure himself enough to be sent home borders on suicidal behavior. Where do suicide and attempted suicide fit into our search for the ways folklore helps warriors deal with the stress and trauma of living and working and fighting in the combat zone?

Suicide is a permanent solution to PTSD, and the US military has been dealing with an "epidemic" of suicides among its active members and veterans since the outset of the wars in Iraq and Afghanistan. A US soldier is "more likely to die by suicide . . . than from combat, accident, or illness" (Rotunda and Freilich 2014, 425). And every day roughly twenty veterans commit suicide (Shane and Kime 2016; Steinhauer 2019). "A Defense Department survey of nearly 30,000 active duty service members from every branch," write Rotunda and Freilich (2014, 422), "revealed that a staggering 2% of Army, 2.3% of Marines, and 3% of Navy respondents had attempted suicide at some point in their careers." Female veterans commit suicide at six times the rate of non-veteran women (Batley 2015).

One explanation for the epidemic of suicides and attempted suicides is the high rate of PTSD in active service members and veterans, one in five of whom experience symptoms that interfere with their everyday lives. This rate means that there are hundreds of thousands of veterans suffering some significant level of symptoms of PTSD.

This discussion of self-harm, attempted suicide, and successful suicide may seem to have wandered far from our interest in folklore as a resource for dealing with the stress and trauma of living, working, and fighting in the combat zone. We have introduced these topics, though, because these behaviors clearly are forms of the "deep play" Geertz (1973) describes, play with stakes so high that it seems irrational to engage in such play. Death is a high stake, certainly, but these behaviors by active military risk court martial proceedings and the potential for a less-than-honorable discharge.

And more generally, we might see the culture of pain in the military, a prominent element in the folklore of the military group, as a therapeutic response to anxiety and trauma. The link between these forms of non-lethal self-harm in the military and relief from the symptoms of PTSD might be seen most clearly in the risky behavior researchers find in veterans, risky behavior that surely counts as deep play.

DEEP PLAY WITH BODY PARTS

Other examples of deep play pose only indirect danger to the player(s) and reflect a darker side of human nature. "Playing" with the bodies of slain enemies or slain civilians on the battlefield is risky because it is officially forbidden and could lead to punishment, including discharge by a court martial. Yet, evidence of warriors' play with the bodies and body parts of enemy combatants can be found everywhere in warriors' memoirs, certainly as far back as WWII.

The American public became aware of this sort of "deep play" with the leaking in 2012 of a video taken by a Marine in Helmond Province, Afghanistan, of his fellow Marines urinating on a pile of the dead bodies of Taliban fighters they had just slain (see Wallis 2012; Mechling 2014). The video sparked public grief and outrage that our Marines would do such a thing; Congress investigated the behavior and some Marines were punished, but the video raises two important questions. First, how common is the desecration of enemy bodies by American warriors, and second, why did a Marine take this video and keep it for later viewing?

From the evidence from warriors' memoirs, we would say that the desecration of enemy bodies has been common in wars (Hedges 2002, 30). Americans like to think of their warriors as noble and incapable of such acts, but the evidence says otherwise. Although "pissing" (we revert here to the folk term for urination) on the bodies of enemy combatants in the 2012 video may seem like an aberration invented by that squad of Marines, in fact there are strong associations between males' pissing on people and things and the expression of masculinity, including male bonding (Mechling 2014). A WWII memoir by Eugene B. Sledge recalls a Martine officer who, whenever he needed to take a piss, would "locate a Japanese corpse, stand over it, and urinate in its mouth" (quoted in Belkin 2012, 126). Cameron's book on the First Marine Division, 1941–1951, reports how common it was for the Marines in the Pacific theater to collect ears and bones as "trophies" (1994, 2, 126).

The 2012 video from Helmond Province landed when Americans were still absorbing a 2011 *Rolling Stone* article by Mark Boal chronicling the murder of Afghan civilians by warriors from Bravo Company (Boal 2011). Some members of Bravo Company took and saved digital photographs of the bodies of the civilians they had killed, and Boal provides this especially disturbing account of the Americans' playing with the dead body of an unarmed, nonthreatening fifteen-year-old Afghan boy, Gul Mudin, they had killed:

> Holding a cigarette rakishly in one hand, Holmes [the Pfc who killed the boy] posed for the camera with Mudin's bloody body and half-naked corpse, grabbing the boy's head by the hair as if it were a trophy deer. . . .
>
> Gibbs started "messing around with the kid," moving his arms and mouth and "acting like the kid was talking." Then, using a pair of razor-sharp medic's shears, he reportedly sliced off the dead boy's pinky finger and gave it to Holmes, as a trophy for killing his first Afghan. . . .
>
> According to his fellow soldiers, Holmes took to carrying the finger with him in a zip-lock bag. "He wanted to keep the finger forever and wanted to dry it out," one of his friends would later report. "He was proud of his finger." (Boal 2011, 4)

Wallis (2012) uses the phrase, "digital trophies," to understand the functions for the warriors of the digital photographs and videos the American warriors take, keep, and share with other warriors. And just as hunters keep animal parts and photographs of killed game as complementary trophies of the hunt (Mechling 2004), so these American warriors are keeping both digital photographs and actual body parts of enemy soldiers as trophies of the experience of battle (see, also, O'Connell 2012, 46). Boal (2011, 14) notes that the members of Bravo Company were keeping pieces of skulls and teeth as trophies. Wallis did not witness the collection of body parts as trophies during his two tours of duty in Iraq, but he understands that "the compulsion to play with these bodies and to take trophies was real and acted upon" (2012, 29).

In a single paragraph is his memoir of a year (May 1969–July 1970) as an infantryman and then helicopter door gunner in Vietnam, John Nesser recounts a sight that is the sort of deep play we mean. His platoon came across some shallow graves of North Vietnamese Army (NVA) soldiers recently killed in an artillery barrage. After digging up the "waxy-looking" corpses, already bloating in death, the deep play began:

> Several soldiers had propped up one of the bodies and had placed a cigarette in the dead man's mouth. Another body had been decapitated by a large chunk of shrapnel and was sprawled near the excavated grave. The mangled head had been placed on a stake in front of the grave as a warning to other NVA. The sight was absolutely ghastly, and it is still vividly etched in my memory. (Nesser 2008, 73)

The severed head on a stake is a very old form of deep play on the battlefield, and we know from war memoirs that deep play with human skulls goes back at least as far as WWI and probably much farther back in the human history of war. Oring (2012) notes the role of human skulls as a "totem" for American troops, and he illustrates his article with a photograph from a Vietnam veteran friend showing a human skull mounted on a stick. Oring's friend told him that the platoon in Vietnam would carry the skull around (sometime in 1969–1970), named the skull "Bruce," and sometimes dressed the skull-on-a-stick in a hat, sunglasses, and pants (Oring 2012). Mechling has in his collection of vintage snapshots a few examples of skulls placed on sticks placed outside a tent or other combat zone shelter (see figure 2.1). McJunkin and Crace's (1983) volume of photographs taken in country in Vietnam includes a photo of a human skull perched upon a stick and wearing a helmet ("The Sentry," FOB Bandit II, November 1970). Wallis points to the case of Marine Sergeant Sanick Dela Cruz, who, in his testimony in the trial of Marne Staff Sergeant Frank Wuterich as the leader of a squad that killed twenty-four unarmed Iraqis in the 2005 "Haditha Massacre," admitted to taking part in the massacre and urinating on the skull of one of the dead Iraqis (Wallis 2012).

The risky deep play with human skulls taps larger cultural and historical meanings of skulls as reminders of our mortality. Hamlet's musing on the skull of "poor Yorick" certainly is one of the best known examples of this symbolism, but portraiture and other paintings from the sixteenth and seventeenth centuries often included skulls as reminders of death and mortality.

Oring's example of deep play with a skull in his friend's platoon in Vietnam is just one of a number of stories about play with bodies the reader finds in Vietnam war memoirs. In his Vietnam memoir Marlantes (2011, 111) reports that "the kids" in his platoon cut off the ears of dead NVA (North Vietnamese soldiers) as trophies of their kills. "The ears went into rubber bands on their helmets or were hung by string around their necks," writes Marlantes; he made them throw away the ears. One of the Vietnam veterans in Lifton's "rap group" in the early 1970s reported seeing a troop carrier with "about twenty human ears tied to the antenna" (1973, 44). Deep in one of the tunnels used by the Vietcong,

J. Ward (1991, 125–26) and another soldier come across a dying female fighter dying from wounds from the grenade they tossed into the tunnel; they pull her dying body from the tunnel and the "weirded-out grunt" with Ward "pulled her pants down and forced a pop-up flare into her vagina and gave it a kick. Her abdomen instantly swelled, and her whole stomach burst open like a volcano with fire and smoke gushing out. God, was there no limit?" One of the Vietnam veterans interviewed by Allan Young told him a series of horrifying stories without showing any emotions; the Marine described to Young the game of "body race," in which the Marines would gather up the dead bodies of North Vietnamese soldiers after a battle, smash the pelvises and spines of the Vietnamese bodies, tie them into balls, and roll them down the hill in a "body race"; when Young asked him if that "game" could be called an atrocity, the Marine matter-of-factly said no (Young 1995, 155). And echoing Nesser's testimony, Webb (1978, 61) describes a Marine putting a cigarette in the mouth of a dead Vietcong combatant for pictures, a scene reminiscent of a scene in the film, *Full Metal Jacket* (1987). Sites (2013, 167) describes the crucifixion of enemy soldiers.

Some of these events belong equally to the "black humor" category. How else should one categorize a warrior's pretending to gnaw at a human femur when presented with a bag full of body parts (Finkel 2013, 61)? Surely real or pretended cannibalism on the battlefield is a form of deep play, but it also shares with black humor the "and there it is" irony in the face of absurdity.

Lifton has written about the psychology of survivors of some of the most traumatic events humans experience (such as the atomic bombing of Hiroshima). Based on his conversations with a "rap group" composed of veterans active in Vietnam Veterans Against the War, his book, *Home from The War* (1973) brings to the attention of readers the traumatic experiences of our warriors and the price they paid. Lifton's analysis is very useful for our purposes because he sees the socialization of boys and young men and the American mythologies of violence as central to both the dysfunctional behavior of the American warriors in the combat zone and their problems when they get home. Lifton was writing his book at about the time the medical profession was recognizing PTSD as a genuine syndrome that needed a clear diagnostic list of symptoms and clear suggestions for therapeutic interventions. Lifton is especially interested in the My Lai massacre and the psychology of atrocity, our next peek into the heart of deep play.

DEEP PLAY—ATROCITIES

As we move our analysis from dark play, like gallows humor, through deep play involving self-harm and play with body parts, we now reach the most troubling form of deep play by warriors—war atrocities. Understandably, calling an atrocity a form of "play" may seem perverse or grotesque, neither play nor folklore, but in thinking and reading about atrocities we feel justified including atrocities as a form of self-therapy. It joins the rank of other terrible, dysfunctional, self-destructive forms of self-help, including drug use and alcohol. We take no pleasure in discussing atrocities (violence against others) as a form of folk therapy alongside violence against self as another form of folk therapy, but there it is.

In his work with Vietnam veterans, therapist Jonathan Shay recognizes that the "berserk state" associated with war atrocities has deep roots in human history. Shay (1994) and others point to Achilles's explosions of violence in *The Iliad* as one of the earliest examples of the berserk state in a warrior. In fact, the reader's theater project, "Theatre of War," performs Sophocles's *Ajax and Philoctetes* for veterans groups and conduct post-performance discussions with the veterans about the age-old experiences of the berserk state in battle (Doerries 2015).

Shay (1994) focuses on the relationship between grief and rage in his writing about the PTSD he treats in the Vietnam veterans he sees." I believe," he writes, "that the emergence of rage out of intense grief is a biological universal and that long-term obstruction of grief and failure to communalize grief can lock a person into chronic rage" (Shay 1994, 54–55). Usually, warriors in the combat zone medicate their grief with drugs and alcohol (1994, 62–63). Our point here, of course, is that the warriors also have available to them a range of folk practices for "self-help" in the face of grief, depression, and rage.

Shay devotes an entire chapter of his 1994 book to the berserk state. He sees six "prompts" for the berserk state in the combat zone. First is "betrayal, insult, or humiliation by a leader" (Shay 1994, 80). The second is "death of a friend-in-arms" (80), precisely what sent Achilles into the berserk state. Third is being wounded. Fourth is "being overrun, surrounded, or trapped." Fifth is "seeing dead comrades who have been mutilated by the enemy." And sixth is "unexpected deliverance from certain death." Shay (82) provides a long list of the symptoms of the berserk state, including "socially disconnected," enraged, cruel, inattentive to own safety, cold, indifferent and reckless. Shay (98) points to a late 1980s survey that reports that 40 percent of Vietnam veterans had engaged in violent acts three or more times in the previous year, a sure symptom of PTSD.

Theweleit (1989) brings a psychoanalytic perspective to his analysis of the psychological states of men in battle. His goal is to understand how the German fixation on the strong male body made it possible for the Nazis to act in cruel ways. He writes about "blackouts" (1989, 164–65), states that can be as benign as fainting or as serious as what Shay (1994) and others call "the berserk state" (Theweleit 1989, 164–65). He makes a great deal of the similarity between blackouts and orgasms (1989, 166,

193, 195), relying in the psychoanalytic insights of Ferenczi, among others. This connection echoes the point he and others make that combat and sex give rise to the same physiological and, accordingly, psychological feelings. Both activities result in "ecstasy," a stepping out from ordinary reality into a state—like Flow (Csikszentmihalyi 1975)—where the subject loses all sense of time and space.

Whether called berserk or blackout states, these states of mind and body fit our argument because the berserk state is an extreme version of the physiological and mental states of warriors who face danger and experience the fight-or-flight moment.

Vietnam veteran Karl Marlantes (2011) uses Jung's notion of "the shadow" in each of us to explore the relationships between shadow, rage, repression, and atrocity. Marlantes, like other war memoirists, shares with the reader the unpleasant news that combat is exhilarating, even sexually arousing, that warriors find "primal pleasure" in killing (30). "What's scary," he writes, "is that it is far easier to take the path of transcendence through destruction than to take the path of transcendence through creation" (63). The transcendent state he refers to here is, in our terms, that state of Flow experienced in combat ("the crack cocaine of all excitement highs," 160). "The transcendent state is a major reason war is an intractable human problem and so difficult to put a stop to. It offers us raw life, vibrant, terrifying, and full blast" (233). Parnell believes it was their "bloodlust" following the witnessing the horror of combat that "bonded the platoon" (2012, 117).

Psychohistorian Robert Jay Lifton sees three different patterns of rage and violence (1973, 137–55). The first is a sense in some veterans that there is a "monster" or "beast" inside them, a feeling similar to the "shadow" Marlantes writes about. The second is rage and violence over the theme of "betrayal," a source of rage that interests Lifton in a number of ways. This sense of rage explains the custom of "fragging" and otherwise killing an officer who is seen as creating unnecessary risk and danger for his men.

Lifton (1973) devotes an entire chapter to the infamous My Lai Massacre, which occurred in that South Vietnamese village (and in a nearby village, My Khe) in March of 1968. In this atrocity a few dozen US soldiers gang-raped, murdered, and mutilated the bodies of hundreds of villagers. The soldiers of Charlie Company arrived in the villages having endured many of the experiences of the sort Shay and others discuss as precursors of the berserk state. The Tet Offensive had taken place two months earlier with many American casualties, and over those months Charlie Company had lost forty comrades dead or wounded, including a well-liked sergeant killed by a land mine.

These experiences are no excuse for the grand scale of killing and mayhem Charlie Company brought to the hamlet of My Lai, of course, but as Americans tried to understand how "American boys" could commit such crimes, these precursors to the berserk state became a main part of the story. After a tangle of coverups and excuses, the army finally held a court martial for twenty-six members of Charlie Company, but only Lt. William Calley, Jr., actually "served time" for the crimes he committed.

Lifton sees not just the immediate three months' stressful and traumatic experiences of Charlie Company as creating the berserk state and the atrocities of My Lai. Like Shay after him, Lifton sees a severe "moral injury" inflicted on the Vietnam warriors. The interviews by Lifton and others found that most Vietnam veterans had serious doubts about the morality of the war and felt deeply the "absurd evil" (Lifton 1973, 37) of the war. The veterans in his "rap group" told stories about the horrors of combat, including the sort of mutilation of enemy bodies we found in memoirs (37). The romantic views of war that the Vietnam veterans grew up with, romantic views we described in chapter 1 on mythologies of masculinity and violence on American popular culture, collided with "the reality of degradation and unspeakable suffering they have witnessed" (38). Recall that American mythologies of masculinity and violence, especially the American Monomyth, satisfy the consumers of the story because the violence is redemptive, leads to a positive state. Lifton knows Campbell's Monomyth and observes that the Vietnam warriors experienced the "test" of manhood, but the arc of the myth is not complete. There is no redemptive moment. This makes for an "atrocity-producing situation," writes Lifton (41).

Instead of the violence leading to redemption and a mature masculinity, the violence at My Lai led it the opposite. "One met the test," writes Lifton, "and stamped out inner doubt by carrying out the most extreme moral inversion and seeing the whole thing to the end. There was both compulsion and satisfaction in doing so" (Lifton 1973, 53). The veterans reported "a need to explode," and their violent acts temporarily relieved that need; the veterans even compared that buildup and release to masturbation (53), and Lifton notes that the rape-murders committed at My Lai took the masturbatory imagery to a new level (53–4).

A sometimes overlooked aspect of the My Lai Massacre is the fact that a few American warriors there refused to participate and even prevented more killing. It took some years for a helicopter crew, labeled "traitors" by members of Congress and the public, to be recognized for their attempts to protect the women and children during the massacre, and Lifton is especially interested in understanding the soldier he calls "the My Lai Survivor," one member of Charlie Company who refused to take part in the slaughter (57). Here is how Lifton accounts for that soldier's refusal. "While it is difficult to know exactly why he was able to join the handful of men who stepped out of the norm and did not participate in the firing," he writes,

> three long-standing psychological patterns seemed significant. First, he had sensitive access to guilt on the basis of particularly strong feelings of right and wrong imbued by family and by protracted Catholic religious training. Second, his lifelong inclination to be a loner, to engage in activities that kept him both physically and psychically separated from others, helped him to maintain a certain degree of autonomy from group influence and from the atrocity-producing situation itself. Third, he had an unusually strong sense of military pride and identification, a form of warrior ethos stressing honor; in Vietnam, and especially at My Lai, he felt both the code and himself to be violated. (58)

A strong sense of right and wrong policed by a strong sense of guilt, the ability to act as an autonomous individual apart from the crowd, and an especially strong sense of pride in the military ethos—these are the qualities of the American Monomythic hero.

There were, as we saw, many individual incidents of deep play by American warriors in Iraq and Afghanistan, and we have drawn just a sample from the memoirs. But if there is a "My Lai moment" in the war in Iraq, surely it was the ongoing atrocities committed by American soldiers, CIA operatives, and private contractors at Abu Ghraib prison, two kilometers west of Baghdad, which had been an infamous prison under the Saddam Hussein regime and became equally infamous when the Americans took over the prison for the detention of terrorist suspects and fighters captured in the war. Although there were signs in 2003 that US authorities were engaged in systematic torture of prisoners at Abu Ghraib, on April 28, 2004, CBS News's *60 Minutes* broadcast a story about abuse within the prison, accompanied by snapshots taken by the abusers themselves. Like the Marines in the earlier Helmond Province episode of urinating on dead Taliban soldiers, the warriors captured their behavior on video and still photos as "digital trophies" (Wallis 2012) of their very masculine domination of the enemy males. Two days after the *60 Minutes* story, veteran war correspondent Seymour Hersh (who won the 1970 Pulitzer Prize for exposing the My Lai massacre and coverup) published a story about the prison, first on the *New Yorker* magazine blog and then in print in the May 10th issue (Hersh 2004). The torture, apparently approved by the government, involved several cruel and painful methods, all chronicled in books about the episode (e.g., Greenberg and Dratel 2005; Gourevitch and Morris 2008; E. Morris 2011) and in a memoir by one of the contract torturers, Eric Fair (2016).

Although the My Lai massacre unfolded over a number of hours, while still satisfying the description of "the berserk state" for therapists and historians, the Abu Ghraib sexual assault, torture, and murder atrocities unfolded over days, weeks, and months. The "berserk state" does not seem to fit the psychological condition that led Americans to treat their human prisoners with such brutal cruelty. If the My Lai massacre was a "hot blood" atrocity, then surely the torture and murders at Abu Ghraib unfolded as a slow-motion "cold blood" atrocity.

Actually, the war memoirs document many "cold blood" atrocities. William March's 1933 novel/memoir of WWI relates the decision to kill unarmed German prisoners of war (POWs) rather than take them back behind American lines. Dixon (2016, 211) describes the killing of unarmed POWs in Vietnam, and Clark (1984, 188) observes the "mercy killing" of a wounded Vietnamese woman. These "cold blood atrocities" appear to weigh just as heavily, if not more so, on the consciences of the veterans writing the memoirs.

FEMALE WARRIORS AND DEEP PLAY

The participation by two female soldiers—Lynndie England and Sabrina Harman—in the Abu Ghraib atrocities raises for us the gender question we have asked and tried to answer with little evidence in each chapter of this book. Do female warriors participate in this particular folk practice, in this case dark play and deep play, and if so does the folk practice serve the same therapeutic goal as it does for the men?

None of the veterans' war memoirs we have read, including those by female warriors, record atrocities by women. We are unable to answer the question we just posed. Our understandable prejudices lead us to believe that women simply do not behave that way. But the Abu Ghraib example challenges that prejudice. We must await more testimony from and about women warriors in the combat zone.

Conclusion

We began this project with the hunch that the folk, the American warriors in the combat zones, had resources in their folk cultures for dealing with the stress and trauma of living, working, and fighting in the combat zone. We thought of this self-help as a form of mental health first-aid, not unlike the short-term, emergency medical assistance provided wounded warriors on the battlefield by medics, corpsmen, and other warriors. Without understanding the medical, scientific reasons why some of their folk practices were providing at least temporary relief from the stress, the warriors settled on some vernacular practices that resemble the therapeutic approaches used by professional mental health practitioners when the veterans get home and seek professional help for dealing with their symptoms of PTSD, especially PET.

We feel confident that the folk practices we have described and analyzed here—adopting companion animals, playfighting, video game play, masturbation, and dark, "deep play"—survive in the folk groups of the warriors because they actually provide some therapeutic relief. We recognize, also, that the folk practices range from the benign to the dangerous and dysfunctional. The abuse of alcohol, other drugs, and seeking risky behavior that could end in injury and even death are not healthy approaches to finding relief from the symptoms of stress.

These few paragraphs have summarized the argument of this book, a wholly appropriate goal for a conclusion. But the conclusion to a book also ought to look forward. Accordingly, we look at what changes in the culture might complicate our argument and we close with brief comments about the possible public policy implications of our study.

THE SOCIAL CONSTRUCTION OF MASCULINITY IN 2019

We began this book with ruminations—both general and specific to our own life histories—on the social construction of normative masculinity in American culture in the last half of the twentieth century, and the generalizations we have made in this book apply to the ideas about manhood young men carried into their service in the twentieth-century wars, especially ideas about the relationship between masculinity and redemptive violence.

Cultures change, though, and we acknowledge that what we have written here about the role of folk cultures of men in small groups might be mere recent history, that changes in both the mythologies of masculinity and changes in the minds of young men (and women) might mean that the structures of heteronormative masculinity are crumbling or, at least, showing signs of crumbling. It is possible that the cumulative effect of the changes—changes in the cultural mythologies of masculinity and violence, changes in the patterns of communication in the small groups wrought by the inclusion of women in the previously all-male combat group, changes in the way the male peer friendship group socializes the boy and young man—might mean, for example, that some aspects of the social construction, maintenance, and repair of masculinity in the military friendship group no longer needs to disguise the homoerotic dimensions of close male bonding, a service performed so well by folklore and its indirection. Perhaps.

Answering these questions about culture change in the twenty-first century and the possible changes in the vernacular folk cultures of male warriors would take a whole other book, but we can map that territory here, ever so briefly.

First, we see little change (as of 2019) in the popular culture narratives featuring the American Monomythic hero and related narratives of the "representative anecdote" based in the American civil religion. In chapter 1 we already cited Lawrence and Jewett (2002) when they point out that the American Monomyth is alive and well and pervasive in the narratives of a great many first-person shooter (FPS) games played by young men and by some young women. Moreover, the many theatrical films featuring various comic book heroes from Marvel appear to critics to be endorsing an "aggressive hypermasculinity," even what has come to be called "toxic masculinity" in an era of the "Me Too" movement and increased awareness of men's large and small aggressions toward women (McIntosh 2015). Monique Jones (2017), writing about the Marvel franchise, invokes an idea that has become central to masculinity studies—namely, that masculinity really is a very fragile construct. "These [Marvel] characters are achetypes for the fragile masculinity that affects too many men in America," she writes. "That fear of not being 'masculine' enough leads to misogyny, self-loathing, fear of homosexuality, and, at its most extreme, the deaths of gay and trans people (usually trans women)" (M. Jones 2017). Jones notes that the print versions of the Marvel stories actually offer a more diverse cast of characters, diverse in their gender and sexuality and ethnicity, but "none of the consideration that goes into Marvel's print stories seem to make it to the film retellings" (M. Jones 2017).

Some media critics have noted a countervailing trend toward more complex masculinities in films (e.g., Roblou 2012). Jack Myers, a notable scholar documenting the lives of Generation Z (born 1996–2020), notes that young men in Gen Z are struggling to define masculinity for themselves, looking to both mass media and social media for clues (Myers 2016, 2017). "Several of today's most popular male figures," writes Myers, "are shaped not by their aggressive, stereotypical take on masculinity, but on other factors altogether: their empathy, kindness and intelligence. There is still a place for 'traditional' masculinity, but it's just one of several options" (Myers 2017).

Interestingly, the business world devoted to marketing and to advising advertisers about the Z Generation as consumers seconds what Myers and other say about the complexity of these young men's ideas about masculinity. While some analysts see a cultural trajectory that might mean the end of "toxic masculinity" (e.g., Keller 2018) in the future, all agree that the messages to young men in both mass media and social media are quite mixed, adding to the confusion and anxiety in the males in Gen Z (West 2018). Despite these views, however, the media culture of FPS games and Marvel heroes seem to us to still be very strong narratives endorsing aggressive masculinity not afraid to use redemptive violence in the name of justice, messages fitting quite well the needs of the military.

Media messages are one thing; the socialization of young men in their peer friendship groups is quite another, for it is not the generic Gen Z male who is recruited by the military but very specific males drawn primarily from particular social classes and ethnic groups, young men who might see the military as a desirable alternative to school or to being unemployed or underemployed in the private sector. That is true for Gen Z women, as well.

This last point plunges us back into the perils of generalization. It is relatively easy to generalize about the shape of the mythological narratives about masculinity and redemptive violence, as we have both narrative analysis and market analysis to bolster our generalizations. Generalizing about the socialization of Gen Z men and women in their peer groups, however, is more difficult, not impossible, but more difficult. We do have some evidence of the groups targeted by military recruiters, and most recently those groups tend to live in poor neighborhoods and attend poor schools (Corcione 2019; Dickstein 2018).

Data made public by the Department of Defense suggests that "most members of the military come from middle-class neighborhoods" (Reynolds and Shendruk 2018). "Among enlisted recruits, 43 percent of men and 56 percent of women are Hispanic or a racial minority. Female recruits are more diverse than the civilian population; they are also more diverse than male recruits" (Reynolds and Shendruk 2018). The number of enlisted women rose from just 2 percent when the draft ended in 1973 to 16 percent (Reynolds and Shendruk 2018).

Reliable numbers on LGBTQ people among the current enlisted personnel are difficult to find, in part because even with the abolition of the "don't ask, don't tell" policy regarding an individual warrior's sexual identity many LGBTQ people have not been eager to declare their sexual orientation or gender identity, and the polices of the Trump administration (especially toward trans people in the military) make people even less enthusiastic to declare themselves lesbian, gay, bisexual, transgender, or queer.

The demographics of current enlisted men and women and the demographics of the populations being aggressively targeted by military recruiters suggest that men entering the military in 2019 *might* hold more traditional ideas about masculinity than would the young men from other populations. We have to say "might" because we do not know. It would be possible to generalize about those recruits if we had actual ethnographic studies of the folk cultures of those male friendship groups, studies which are few and far between. Reporters in the popular press give us snapshots of those being recruited, but we are left with mere speculation about the relation of those male recruits and the scholarly portrait of Gen Z in general.

The gender, ethnic, and even sexual diversity of the current military actually reflects well the demographics and attitudes of recent generations. Twenge (2006, 2017) considers the several proposed names for the generation after the millennials (born 1982–2000) and she settles on her own neologism, the "iGen." For this generation, born in 1995 and thereafter, the defining event in their lives and for the generation was the introduction of the iPhone in 2007, and then the iPad in 2010 (Twenge 2017, 2). The iGen lives many hours a day with and on their handheld devices (on average six hours a day), says Twenge (2017, 51), interacting as much (or more) online than face-to-face. Twenge sees enormous consequences of this life lived online.

Relying on four large sample studies and her own small sample (twenty-three) of interviews with members of the generation (beyond talking with her own students in classes), Twenge devotes a chapter to each of ten characteristics (each beginning with an "i") she sees in the iGen. This generation, for example, is "in no hurry" to grow up (2017, 17–48). This means, to us, that young military recruits may be more likely to be less self-reliant at that age than the same-age cohort from earlier generations. The iGen are delaying the key signals of adulthood. Other characteristics of the iGen are "insecure," "irreligious," and "independent."

Twenge (2017) identifies a few characteristics, such as "in person no more" and "independent," that combine to paint a picture of members of the iGen as more isolated from their peers than were previous generations at the same age. As folklorists we are a bit skeptical about that conclusion from survey data because we suspect that young men still have lots of socializing experiences in the male friendship group, from Scout troops and sports teams to informal gatherings at school and in homes. We see nothing to indicate that when they join the military the young men of the iGen will have a deficit of understanding the dynamics of the male friendship group, including the stylized aggression found in the group. Basic training (boot camp), in any event, cements the identification of the individual with the group. This is not to say that recruits do not carve out time for individual expressions of identity and resistance, a topic we are writing about in a separate project. We observe here, simply, that the independence and experience of doing things alone (if being online counts as "alone," which it does not) in the iGen seems to us unlikely to change the dynamics of men in groups in the military.

The iGen recruit's possible expectation of more privacy is destroyed by the basic training experience, and judging from the war memoirs by younger men, anyway, we would expect no change in the male warrior's talking about and joking about masturbation as a way to relieve stress in the combat zone. The ubiquity of porn on their handheld devices is now an established element in the sexuality of the iGen.

Twenge (2017) relies mainly on the four large sample studies in making her generalizations about the iGen, and her interviews do not dwell much on gender differences, but a few patterns might suggest some interesting changes for women who join what is still a very masculine culture, the military. Earlier we mentioned the fact that ethnographers have observed over the years that girls' play is becoming more like boys' play, and that Title IX (1972) created something of a revolution in gender by giving young women access to team sports and to what young men learn in that framed play.

If Twenge is right, then both men and women in the iGen are likely to believe that gender identity is "fluid," not fixed. And the same fluidity can be found in the iGen views of sexual identity. Put differently, we might expect that women in the military themselves have less-stereotyped views of gender and sexuality, and the men they join in the military might be less rigid in their own views of gender identity and sexual identity.

We do not want to overstate this case. So many biological and social pressures in the male friendship group favor traditional American views of normative heterosexual masculinity. We expect, for example, that the need for a young man to "prove" his masculinity by passing daily "tests"—from being able to take a joke to braving combat—is still a dynamic in the male friendship group. At the same time, the strong homoerotic elements of some of the folklore, especially the R&T playfighting, doubtless takes on more complicated meanings if the men present are openly gay, bisexual, or even trans men, which is now possible in the military. Both men and women in the iGen have positive attitudes about sexual fluidity (Twenge 2017, 227–35).

Twenge's book, unfortunately, is not very good about distinguishing the poor kids from the middle-class kids. The large national studies she draws upon doubtless contain some working-class youth, and as a California State University (San Diego) professor she doubtless has students drawn from a range of economic and social circumstances. Necessarily Twenge faces our dilemma, that of making useful generalizations, but a few of the things we would like to know about the young men targeted for military recruitment simply are not answered by her work. For example, do the recruits share typical iGen or Gen Z attitudes about the "fluidity" ethnic and sexual identity?

Here, then, are the cultural changes at play as we think about the ways the vernacular practices of warriors might help them cope with the stresses of living, working, and fighting in the combat zone. The new male recruit likely has consumed a diet of mass media narratives endorsing an "aggressive masculinity." He likely comes from social and economic peer groups that hold more traditional views of masculinity, views that might see misogyny and homophobia as acceptable strategies for "proving" one's manhood. As for the female warriors, everything about iGen points to a continuation of their becoming more and more like men in the details of their interactions in their folk, friendship groups.

PUBLIC POLICY IMPLICATIONS

In the spirit of C. Wright Mills, whom we cited at the outset of this book as an advocate of the reflexive study of American culture as an exercise in "connecting private troubles with public issues" (Mills 1959), we offer here a few suggestions about the implications of our study for public policy, especially policy laid down by the military authorities.

As we saw in our chapter on the adoption of animals, especially dogs, in the combat zone, the military is moving slowly toward letting warriors bring back home the animals they adopt when abroad. Similarly, the military's strict regulations about masturbation can be relaxed, should be relaxed, always keeping in mind mission readiness and unit cohesion.

The military establishment has nothing against FPS video games; indeed, as we saw, the military develops such games as an element of its marketing and recruitment of young people, especially young men. The attack on FPS games comes from outside the military. Whenever there is a mass murder shooting event, such as the murder of students and teachers on Valentine's Day, 2018, at Parkland High School in Florida, there is what historians call a "moral panic" about FPS video games. President Trump leaped to blaming video games for that mass murder, despite overwhelming evidence that there is no link between playing the games and becoming violent (Werner 2018). If we are right in our assessment of the positive outcomes for players of FPS games, including the benefits of imagining one's own death, then the attempts in the public sphere to ban those games would be a mistake.

Perhaps the only policy implication from our study of "deep play" in the combat zone has to do with the military's policy on accepting young men and women who have physical evidence of self-harm (e.g., cutting, branding). Even this policy is softening a bit, as the military will accept those people if they can provide testimony from a therapist that they are not a threat to themselves or others.

There is one larger "public policy" question worth mentioning in conclusion. For that we return to Robert Jay Lifton's very thoughtful book about the Vietnam War and its veterans. *Home from the War* (1973). When Lifton interviewed the one member of the platoon who did not participate in the My Lai Massacre, Lifton wanted to know what reservoir of strength made it possible for that individual to refrain from participating. It turns out that the soldier's strong sense of honor was the key; to participate in the atrocity would be dishonorable.

Near the end of his wise book Lifton offers some thoughts on honor. He urges his fellow Americans to dislodge "the individual and collective sense of honor from the warrior ethos" (1973, 376–77). "For rather than fly in the face of biology or evolution," he continues, "the transformation we are discussing would call upon a full store of manly and womanly virtue, of male bonding (and possibly female bonding as well), but around forms other than those of the warrior ethos" (377). As in his other work, Lifton endorses a sense of immortality disconnected from violence and destruction.

Gibson's (1994) analysis of the rise of a new warrior culture in the 1980s ends with a recommendation resembling Lifton's. Gibson recognizes the tremendous power of "enchantment" in the socialization of young men. "Rethinking parenting and recasting initiation rites will no doubt move us toward a new masculine ideal," he writes, "but they will not break the spell of warrior dreams unless we recognize something even more basic. At the broadest level, paramilitary culture shows the continuing need for myth and ritual even in the heart of the modern secular world" (306). The socialization of boys, in other words, needs to reject the "enchantment" of paramilitary culture and invent new initiation rites and institutions for the "reenchantment" of mature adulthood. Such new initiation rites and institutions combine an "extraordinary level of adventure and the experience of community" (307).

Jay notes at this point, not surprisingly, that the Boy Scouts can provide enchanted initiation to both young men and young women (newly admitted in 2019), but that is only one example of an institution that might design initiation into manhood without thinking that aggression and violence have to be part of that transition.

More than one commentator has noted that "adventure" and "community" are what veterans miss most in the transition from the military to civilian life. When you read as many war memoirs as we have for this book, you encounter many vivid descriptions of what happens to young men when their "warrior dreams" meet the reality of war. Gibson (1994) writes that the mythology of "regeneration through violence" broke in the defeat in Vietnam (10), but it is clear from memoirs even from earlier wars that the cynicism born of combat experience kills forever any romantic notion of proving one's manhood through the test of fire.

A common motif in war memoirs of the Gulf War and the wars in Iraq and Afghanistan, wars without a draft and relying on recruiting, is that the recruiting officer "lied" in promising everything from the job specialty in service to the place where posted. We might just as easily talk about the culture's "lie" to young men, a lie embodied in the mythology of the comic books, the movies, the television shows, and the video game narratives he consumed from an early age.

As culture critics, we want to acknowledge as well the effects upon warriors and veterans of the shattering of the American mythologies of masculinity and violence. Many of the memoirs we have read for this book convey the blow to the young man's sense of himself when the irrationality of war becomes clear to him. That irrationality enters some of the vernacular genres we analyze here, from gallows humor to dark play. The absolute irrationality and contingency of combat undermines the mythology of the regeneration of masculinity through violence, often leaving the warrior with the feeling he was a fool for ever believing the mythology.

The further import of the destruction of the American Monomyth and its relatives in American mythology lies in the warrior's return home. Recall that the American Monomythic hero, who restores the balance of safety and peace to the community, finally cannot be absorbed by the community precisely because of his talent for violence. Shane must ride off into the sunset, Rambo must walk off into the jungle, Superman can never lead a normal life.

Many male veterans report feelings of impotence upon their return to civilian life. In the military—especially in combat roles—the warriors experienced a level of power they never experienced in everyday civilian life. The weapons they carry are capable of great violence; the warrior is a demi-god, dispensing death and deciding in many cases who lives and who dies. Suddenly, upon leaving military service, the veteran wields none of that power.

To write about honor in the closing paragraphs of this book on folklore and PTSD may seem odd to the reader, but we both have a strong sense of honor, for JP a sense of honor honed in the Marine Corps and for Jay a sense of honor honed in the Boy Scouts. To write about honor may seem old-fashioned, as the concept has its roots in the nineteenth century and earlier. One of the great transformations in American culture was the change from talk about "character" (the context giving meaning to "honor") to talk about "personality," a transformation evident by the first decade of the twentieth century (Susman 1985). Jay notes here that the

Boy Scouts of America was founded in 1910. And when there was a revival of interest in "character education" in the Reagan 1980s (Hunter 2000), the discussion seemed politically conservative and masculine, doubtless a symptom of the same sense of loss of white male privilege that fueled the mythopoetic men's movement at the same time.

The concept of honor plays no role in either Twenge's 2017 book on the iGen nor her 2006 book on the narcissism of the millennial generation. This does not mean that the sense of honor in young people is dead, nor does it mean that we cannot forge a renewed concept of honor and character along the lines proposed by Lifton in 1973, or forge initiation rituals that capture the enchantment of adventure and community without redemptive violence. Young people still are Scouts, and young people still are attracted to the military for its promise of belonging and a purpose larger than the individual. Public policy can be steered toward building and supporting institutions for the socialization of boys without linking honor and enchantment to aggressive masculinity, and public policy can make it easier for veterans and for those who serve them to create experiences easing the transition from the adventure and bonding of combat to the adventure and bonding of friendship in civilian life.

References

Abrams, David. n.d. "Reading in Iraq—One Soldier's Devotion to Books." Abe Books blog https://www.abebooks.com/docs/Community/Featured/soldiers-devotion-full.shtml#full. Last accessed May 1, 2019.

Adler, Patricia A., and Peter Adler. 2011. *The Tender Cut: Inside the Hidden World of Self-Injury*. New York: New York University Press.

Allen, Robertson. 2017. *America's Digital Army: Games at Work and War*. Lincoln, NE: University of Nebraska Press.

Ambrose, Stephen E. 1992. *Band of Brothers*. New York: Simon and Schuster.

Ancelet, Barry Jean, Marcia Gaudet, and Carl Lindahl, eds. 2013. *Second Line Rescue: Improvised Responses to Katrina and Rita*. Jackson, MS: University Press of Mississippi.

Arluke, Arnold, and Lauren Rolfe. 2013. *The Photographed Cat: Picturing Human-Feline Ties, 1890–1940*. Syracuse, NY: Syracuse University Press.

Bancroft, J. 2005. "The Endocrinology of Sexual Arousal." *Journal of Endocrinology* 186:411–27. http://joe.endocrinology-journals.org/content/186/3/411.full. Last accessed May 11, 2019.

Baritz, Loren. 1985. *Backfire: A History of How American Culture Led Us into Vietnam and Made Us Fight the Way We Did*. New York: William Morrow & Co.

Bateson, Gregory. 1972 [1955]. "A Theory of Play and Fantasy." In *Steps to an Ecology of Mind*, 177–93. New York: Ballantine.

———. 1979. *Mind and Nature: A Necessary Unity*. New York: E.P. Dutton.

Batley, Melanie. 2015. "Suicide Rates Among Female Vets 'Obscenely High': Report." Newsmax. http://www.newsmax.com/Newsfront/veterans-women-military-suicide/2015/06/11/id/650051/. Last accessed May 11, 2019.

Beck, Julie. 2015. "What Good Is Thinking About Death?" *The Atlantic* blog May 28. https://www.theatlantic.com/health/archive/2015/05/what-good-is-thinking-about-death/394151/. Last accessed May 1, 2019.

Beetz, Andrea, et al. 2012. "Psychosocial and Psychophysiological Effects of Human-Animal Interactions: The Possible Role of Oxytocin." *Frontiers in Psychology* https://www.ncbi.nlm.nih.gov/pmc/articles/PMC3408111/. Last accessed May 11, 2019.

Belkin, Aaron. 2012. *Bring Me Men: Military Masculinity and the Benign Façade of American Empire, 1898–2001*. New York: Columbia University Press.

Bellah, Robert. 1967. "Civil Religion in America." *Daedalus* 96: 1–21.

Ben-Amos, Dan. 1971. "Toward a Definition of Folklore in Context." *Journal of American Folklore* 84: 3–15.

Beneke, Timothy. 1997. *Proving Manhood: Reflections on Sex and Sexism*. Berkeley, CA: University of California Press.

Berger, Peter L. and Thomas Luckmann. 1967. *The Social Construction of Reality: A Treatise on the Sociology of Knowledge*. Garden City, NY: Anchor Doubleday.

Beresin, Anna R. 2010. *Recess Battles: Playing, Fighting, and Storytelling*. Jackson, MS: University Press of Mississippi.

Best, Joel. 1990. *Threatened Children: Rhetoric and Concern about Child Victims*. Chicago: University of Chicago Press.

Bettelheim, Bruno. 1954. *Symbolic Wounds: Puberty Rites and the Envious Male*. New York: Free Press.

Biank, Tanya. 2013. *Undaunted: The Real Story of America's Servicewomen in Today's Military*. New York: New American Library.

Boal, Mark. 2011. "The Kill Team: How U.S. Soldiers in Afghanistan Murdered Innocent Civilians." *Rolling Stone* March 27. https://www.rollingstone.com/politics/politics-news/the-kill-team-how-u-s-soldiers-in-afghanistan-murdered-innocent-civilians-169793/. Last accessed May 11, 2019.
Bordo, Susan. 1999. *The Male Body: A New Look at Men in Public and in Private*. New York: Farrar, Straus and Giroux.
Borelli, Lizette. 2014. "Brain on Sex: How the Brain Functions During an Orgasm." Medical Daily. http://www.medicaldaily.com/brain-sex-how-brain-functions-during-orgasm-274052. Last accessed May 11, 2019.
Boston Women's Health Book Collective. 1973. *Our Bodies, Ourselves: A Book by and for Women*. New York: Simon and Schuster.
Botvin, G. J., and Brian Sutton-Smith. 1977. "The Development of Structural Complexity in Children's Fantasy Narratives." *Developmental Psychology* 13:377–88.
Bronner, Simon J. 1988, *American Children's Folklore*, annotated edition. Little Rock, AR: August House.
———. 1996. *The Carver's Art: Crafting Meaning from Wood*. Lexington, KY: University Press of Kentucky.
———. 2006. *Crossing the Line: Violence, Play, and Drama in Naval Equator Traditions*. Amsterdam: Amsterdam University Press.
———. 2012. *Campus Traditions: Folklore from the Old-Time College to the Modern Mega-University*. Jackson, MS: University Press of Mississippi.
Burden, Matthew Currier. 2006. *The Blog of War*. New York: Simon and Schuster.
Burghardt, Gordon M. 2005. *The Genesis of Animal Play: Testing the Limits*. Cambridge, MA: MIT Press.
Burke, Carol. 2004. *Camp All-American, Hanoi Jane, and the High-and-Tight: Gender, Folklore, and Changing Military Culture*. Boston: Beacon Press.
Burke, Kenneth. 1973. *The Philosophy of Literary Form: Studies in Symbolic Action*. 3rd ed.; Berkeley, CA: University of California Press.
Burhham, John C. 2008. *A Soldier's Best Friend: Scout Dogs and Their Handlers in the Vietnam War*. New York: Union Square Press.
Burns, Thomas A. 1984. "Doing the Wash: Cycle Two." *Western Folklore* 43: 122–26.
Busch, Benjamin. 2012. *Dust to Dust: A Memoir*. New York: Ecco.
Buzzell, Colby. 2005. *My War: Killing Time in Iraq*. New York: Putnam's Sons.
Cameron, Craig M. 1994. *American Samurai: Myth, Imagination, and the Conduct of Battle in the First Marine Division, 1941–1951*. Cambridge, UK: Cambridge University Press.
Campbell, Joseph. 1949. *The Hero With a Thousand Faces*. New York: Pantheon.
Cannon, Walter Bradford. 1915. *Bodily Changes in Pain, Hunger, Fear, and Rage: An Account of Recent Researches Into the Function of Emotional Excitement*. New York: D. Appleton and Company.
Chodorow, Nancy. 1978. *The Reproduction of Mothering: Psychoanalysis and the Sociology of Gender*. Berkeley, CA: University of California Press.
Clark, Johnnie M. 1984. *Guns Up*! New York: Ballantine.
Cohen, Jennie. 2011. "Assistance Dogs: Learning New Tricks for Centuries." http://www.history.com/news/assistance-dogs-learning-new-tricks-for-centuries Last accessed May 1, 2019.
Colin, Chris. 2012. "How Dogs Can Help Veterans Overcome PTSD." *Smithsonian*. http://www.smithsonianmag.com/science-nature/how-dogs-can-help-veterans-overcome-ptsd-137582968/. Last Accessed May 11, 2019.
Collins, Max Allen. 2000. *For the Boys: The Racy Pin-Ups of World War II*. Portland, OR: Collectors Press.
Corcione, Danielle. 2019. "The Military Targets Youth for Recruitment, Especially at Poor Schools" *Teen Vogue* January 22. https://www.teenvogue.com/story/the-military-targets-youth-for-recruitment. Last accessed May 1, 2019.
Courtwright, David T. 1996. *Violent Land: Single Men and Social Disorder from the Frontier to the Inner City*. Cambridge, MA: Harvard University Press.

Crawford, John. 2005. *The Last True Story I'll Ever Tell: An Accidental Soldier's Account of the War in Iraq*. New York: Riverhead.
Csikszentmihalyi, Mihaly. 1975. *Beyond Boredom and Anxiety*. San Francisco, CA: Jossey-Bass.
Daughtry, J. Martin. 2015. *Listening to War: Sound, Music, Trauma, and Survival in Wartime Iraq*. Oxford, UK: Oxford University Press.
David, D., and R. Brannon, eds. 1976. *The Forty-nine Percent Majority: The Male Sex Role*. Reading, MA: Addison-Wesley.
Delfino, Andrew, and Jay Mechling. 2017. "Wrestling with Masculinity." *Children's Folklore Review* 38: 57–77.
Dickstein, Corey, 2017. "Army: No Waivers for Self-Mutilators, Others with Serious Mental Health Issues." *Stars and Stripes* Nov. 15. https://www.stripes.com/army-no-waivers-for-self-mutilators-others-with-serious-mental-health-issues-1.497975. Last accessed on May 1, 2019.
———. 2018. "Army Targets Young Americans in New Ways for Recruiting." *Stars and Stripes* October 9. https://www.stripes.com/army-targets-young-americans-in-new-ways-for-recruiting-1.551040. Last accessed May 1, 2019.
Dixon, James. 2016. *Things I'll Never Forget: Memories of a Marine in Vietnam*. N.p.: Do Right Press.
Dodson, Betty. 1974. *Liberating Masturbation*. New York: Bodysex Designs.
———. 1987. *Sex for One: The Joy of Self-Loving*. New York: Harmony Books.
Doerries, Bryan. 2015. *The Theater of War: What Ancient Greek Tragedies Can Teach Us Today*. New York: Knopf.
Dokoupil, Tony. 2008. "Soldiers' Self-Harm: Anything Not to Go Back to Iraq." *Newsweek* http://www.newsweek.com/soldiers-self-harm-anything-not-go-back-iraq-90995. Last accessed May 1, 2019.
Douglas, Mary. 1966. *Purity and Danger: An Analysis of Concepts of Pollution and Taboo*. London: Routledge and Kegan Paul.
Driskill, Robert. 2017. *That Close: A Memory of Combat in Vietnam*. N.p.: Independently Published.
Dundes, Alan. 1965. "What Is Folklore?" In *The Study of Folklore,* ed. Alan Dundes. Upper Saddle River, NJ: Prentice-Hall.
———. 1966. "Here I Sit—A Study of American Latrinalia." *Papers of the Kroeber Anthropological Society* 34: 91–105. Reprinted in *The Meaning of Folklore: The Analytical Essays of Alan Dundes,* edited by Simon J. Bronner, 360–74. Logan, UT: Utah State University Press, 2007.
———. 1997. "Traditional Male Combat: From Game to War." In Alan Dundes, *From Game to War and Other Psychoanalytic Essays on Folklore*, 25–45. Lexington, KY: University Press of Kentucky.
Ehrenreich, Barbara. 1997. *Blood Rites: Origins and History of the Passions of War*. New York: Metropolitan Books.
Ethell, Jeffrey L., and Clarence Simonsen. 2003. *The History of Aircraft Nose Art: WW1 to Today*. London: Motorbooks Intl.
Fair, Eric. 2016. *Consequence: A Memoir*. New York: Henry Holt and Co.
Ferenczi, Sandor, Karl Abraham, Ernst Simmel, and Ernest Jones. 1921. *Psycho-Analysis and the War Neuroses*. London: The International Psycho-Analytical Press.
Finkel, David. 2009. *The Good Soldiers*. New York: Picador, Farrar, Straus & Giroux.
———. 2013. *Thank You for Your Service*. New York: Farrar, Straus & Giroux.
Finley, Erin. 2011. *Fields of Combat: Understanding PTSD Among Veterans of Iraq and Afghanistan*. Ithaca, NY: Cornell University Press.
Fogel, Alan. 2010. "Male and Female Orgasm: Not So Different?" *Psychology Today* blog April 16. https://www.psychologytoday.com/blog/body-sense/201004/male-and-female-orgasm-not-so-different. Last accessed May 11, 2019.
Freud, Sigmund. 1922 [1920]. *Beyond the Pleasure Principle*. Trans. C. J. M. Hubback. London: International Psycho-Analytical Press.

———. 1961 [1927]. "Humour." In The *Future of Illusion, Civilization and Its Discontents and Other Works*, Standard Edition Vol. 21, 159–66. London: Hogarth Press.
Friedan, Betty. 1963. *The Feminine Mystique*. New York: Dell.
Friedrich, Brandon. 2017. "This Military-Grade Masturbation Device is Designed to Service Our Troops." *Maxim* May 17. https://www.maxim.com/maxim-man/lifetime-silicone-stroker-2017–5. Last access May 1, 2019.
Frosh, Stephen. 1994. *Sexual Difference: Masculinity and Psychoanalysis*. London: Routledge.
Fuller, Thomas. 2018. "Violence Strikes a Veterans Program that Strove to Prevent It." *New York Times* March 10 https://www.nytimes.com/2018/03/10/us/yountville-veterans-pathway-shooting.html. Last access May 1, 2019.
Gabor, Mark. 1972. *The Pin-Up: A Modest History*. New York: Universe Books.
Garvey, Anna. 2015. "The Oregon Trail Generation: Life Before and After Mainstream Tech." *Social Media Week* https://socialmediaweek.org/blog/2015/04/oregon-trail-generation/. Last accessed May 1, 2019.
Geertz, Clifford. 1973. *The Interpretation of Cultures*. New York: Basic Books.
———. 1983 [1975]. "Common Sense as a Cultural System." In *Local Knowledge*, 73–93. New York: Basic Books.
Gibson, James William. 1994. *Warrior Dreams: Violence and Manhood in Post-Vietnam America*. New York: Hill and Wang.
Gilman, Lisa. 2016. *My Music, My War: The Listening Habits of U.S. Troops in Iraq and Afghanistan*. Middletown, CT: Wesleyan University Press.
Goffman, Erving. 1961. *Asylums: Essays on the Social Situation of Mental Patients and Other Inmates*. Garden City, NY: Anchor Books.
———. 1974. *Frame Analysis*. New York: Harper and Row.
Goldstein, Joshua S. 2001. *War and Gender: How Gender Shapes the War System and Vice Versa*. Cambridge, UK: Cambridge University Press.
Goodman, Katy. 2013. "How Video Games Help Soldiers Deal with the Horrors of War." http://kotaku.com/how-video-games-are-helping-soldiers-deal-with-the-horr-1411559341. Last accessed May 1, 2019.
Goodwin, Marjorie H. 2006. *The Hidden Life of Girls: Games of Stance, Status, and Exclusion*. Malden, MA: Blackwell Publishers.
Goolsby, Jesse. 2015. *I'd Walk With My Friends If I Could Find Them*. Boston: Houghton Mifflin Harcourt.
Gourevitch, Philip, and Erroll Morris. 2008. *Standard Operating Procedure*. New York: Penguin Press.
Goyton, R. 1998. "'Pissing Out the Fire': Reasserting Masculine Identity in a Closure Ritual." *Prized Writing*. Davis, CA: Writing Program, University of California, Davis.
Gray, J. Glenn. 1959. *The Warriors: Reflection on Men in Battle*. New York: Harper & Row.
Greenberg, Karen J., and Joshua L. Dratel, eds. 2005. *The Torture Papers: The Road to Abu Ghraib*. New York: Cambridge University Press.
Grier, Katherine C. 2006. *Pets in America: A History*. Chapel Hil, NC: University of North Carolina Press.
Grinker, R. R., and J. P. Spiegel. 1945. *War Neuroses*. Philadelphia, PA: Blakiston.
Groos, Karl. 1898. *The Play of Animals*. New York: D. Appleton and Co.
Grossman, Dave. 2009. *On Killing: The Psychological Cost of Learning to Kill in War and Society*. New York: Little, Brown and Company.
Grossman, Dave, with Loren W. Christensen. 2008. *On Combat: The Psychology and Physiology of Deadly Conflict in War and Peace*. Np: Warrior Science Publications.
Handelman, Don. 1977. "Play and Ritual: Complementary Frames of Meta-Communication." In *It's a Funny Thing, Humour*, edited by A. J. Chapman and H. C. Foote, 185–92. Oxford, UK: Pergamon.

Healy, Patrick. 2009. "The Anguish of War for Today's Soldiers, Explored by Sophocles." *New York Times* Nov. 11. http://www.nytimes.com/2009/11/12/theater/12greeks.html. Last accessed May 1, 2019.
Hedges, Chris. 2002. *War is a Force That Gives Us Meaning*. New York: Anchor Books.
Hegar, Mary Jennings. 2017. *Shoot Like a Girl: One Woman's Dramatic Fight in Afghanistan and on the Home Front*. New York: New American Library.
Heller, Joseph. 1961. *Catch-22*. New York: Simon & Schuster.
Hersh, Seymour M. 2004. "Torture at Abu Ghraib." *The New Yorker* May 10. https://www.newyorker.com/magazine/2004/05/10/torture-at-abu-ghraib. Last accessed May 1, 2019.
Hetherington, Tim. 2010. *Infidel*. London: ChistBoot Ltd.
Hirschfeld, Magnus. 1941 [1934]. *The Sexual History of the World War*. New York: Cadillac Publishing Co.
Holmes, Emily A., Ella L. James, Thomas Coode-Bate, and Catherine Deeprose. 2009. "Can Playing the Computer Game 'Tetris' Reduce the Build-up of Flashbacks for Trauma? A proposal from Cognitive Science." PLoS ONE 4(1):1–6.
Holmstedt, Kirsten. 2007. *Band of Sisters: American Women at War in Iraq*. Mechanicsburg, PA: Stackpole Books.
———. 2009. *The Girls Come Marching Home: Stories of Women Warriors Returning from the War in Iraq*. Mechanicsburg, PA: Stackpole Books.
Howe, Neil, and Bill Strauss. 1993. *13th Gen: Abort, Retry, Ignore, Fail?* New York: Vintage Books.
Howe, Neil, Bill Strauss, and William Strauss. 2000. *Millennials Rising: The Next Great Generation*. New York: Vintage Books.
Hoyt, Margaret. 2005. "Pinups." In *The Encyclopedia of War and American Society*, edited by Peter Karsten, 632–33. Thousand Oaks, CA: Sage.
Hughes, Linda. 1993. "'You Have to Do It with Style': Girls' Games and Girls' Gaming." In *Feminist Theory and the Study of Folklore*, edited by T. Hollis, L. Pershing, and M.J. Young, 230–48. Urbana, IL: University of Illinois Press.
———. 1999. "Children's Games and Gaming." In *Children's Folklore: A Sourcebook*, edited by B. Sutton-Smith, J. Mechling, T. W. Johnson, and F. R. McMahon, 94–119. Logan, UT: Utah State University Press.
Hunter, James Davison. 2000. *The Death of Character: Moral Education in an Age Without Good or Evil*. New York: Basic Books.
Jackson, Bruce. 1965. "Prison Folklore." *Journal of American Folklore* 310: 317–29.
Jarvis, Christina S. 2010. *The Male Body at War: American Masculinity during World War II*. DeKalb, IL: Northern Illinois University Press.
Jarvis, Pam. 2006. "'Rough and Tumble' Play: Lessons in Life." *Evolutionary Biology* 4: 330–346.
Jeffords, Susan. 1993. *Hard Bodies: Hollywood Masculinity in the Reagan Era*. New Brunswick, NJ: Rutgers University Press.
Jewett, Robert, and John Shelton Lawrence. 1977. *The American Monomyth*. Garden City, NY: Anchor Press/Doubleday.
Jones, Gerard. 2002. *Killing Monsters: Why Children Need Fantasy, Super-Heroes, and Make-Believe Violence*. New York: Basic Books.
Jones, James. 1962. *The Thin Red Line*. New York: Charles Scribner's Sons.
Jones, Monique. 2017. "The Fragile Masculinity of the MCU (Or Why Captain America Shouldn't Be Afraid to Cry)." *Slash Film* August 3. https://www.slashfilm.com/the-fragile-masculinity-of-the-mcu/. Last accessed May 1, 2019.
Jordan, Ellen. 1995. "Fighting Boys and Fantasy Play: The Construction of Masculinity in the Early Years of School." *Gender and Education*, 7: 69–87.
Junger, Sebastian. 2010. *War*. New York: Twelve.
Kardiner, Abram. 1941. *The Traumatic Neuroses of War*. New York: Hoeber.
Keller, Jared. 2018. "The (Coming) End of Toxic Masculinity." *Pacific Standard* January 10. https://psmag.com/social-justice/toxic-masculinity-on-its-way-out Last accessed May 1, 2019.

Kelly, Diane. 2015. "9 Animals that Masturbate (Other Than Humans)." Gizmmodo https://gizmodo.com/9-animals-that-masturbate-other-than-humans-1723592357. Last accessed May 1, 2019.

Kimmel, Michael. 2005. *The Gender of Desire; Essays on Male Sexuality*. Albany, NY: State University of New York Press.

———. 2008. *Guyland: The Perilous World Where Boys Become Men*. New York: Harper.

King, Stephen. 1980. *Danse Macabre*. New York: Berkley.

Kopelman, Jay, with Melinda Roth. 2006. *From Baghdad, With Love: A Marine, the War, and a Dog Named Lava*. Guilford, CT: Lyons Press.

Kovic, Ron. 1976. *Born on the Fourth of July*. New York: McGraw Hill.

Lakoff, George, and Mark Johnson. 1980. *Metaphors We Live By*. Chicago: University of Chicago Press.

Langlois, Janet L. 1991. "'Hold the Mayo': Purity and Danger in an AIDS Legend." *Contemporary Legend* 1(1): 153–172.

Laquer, Thomas W. 2003. *Solitary Sex: The Cultural History of Masturbation*. New York: Zone Books.

Lawrence, John Shelton, and Robert Jewett. 2002. *The Myth of the American Superhero*. Grand Rapids, MI: William B. Eerdmans Publishing Company.

Lemish, Michael G. 1996. *War Dogs: A History of Loyalty and Heroism*. Washington, DC: Brassey's.

———. 2009. *Forever Forward: K-9 Operations in Vietnam*. Atglen, PA: Schiffer Military History.

Lemmon, Gayle Tzemach. 2015. *Ashley's War: The Untold Story of a Team of Women Soldiers on the Special Ops Battlefield*. New York: HarperCollins.

LeVay, Simon. 1993. *The Sexual Brain*. Cambridge, MA: MIT Press.

Levinson, Boris. 1969. *Pet-oriented Child Psychotherapy*. Springfield, IL: Charles C. Thomas, Publisher.

Lewin, Tamar. 2007. "More Girls Take Part in High School Wrestling." *New York Times*, February 17, 2007. www.nytimes.com/2007/02/17/nyregion/17wrestle.html?_r=1&. Last accessed May 1, 2019.

Lewis, R. W. B. 1955. *The American Adam*. Chicago: University of Chicago Press.

Lifton, Robert Jay. 1973. *Home from the War: Vietnam Veterans, Neither Victims nor Executioners*. New York; Basic Books.

———. 1987. *The Future of Immortality and Other Essays for a Nuclear Age*. New York: Basic Books.

Lindahl, Carl. 2012. "Legends of Hurricane Katrina: The Right to be Wrong, Survivor-to-Survivor Storytelling, and Healing." *Journal of American Folklore* 125: 139–76.

Lipman, Steve. 1991. *Laughter in Hell: The Use of Humour During the Holocaust*. Northvale, NJ: Jason Aronson.

Lissman, P. 1919. *Die Wirkungen des Krieges auf das Månnliche Geschlechtsleben* [The Effects of War on the Sex Life of Men]. Munchen.

Lyman, Peter. 1987. "The Fraternal Bond as a Joking Relationship: A Case Study of the Role of Sexist Jokes in Male Group Bonding." In *Changing Men*, edited by Michael Kimmel, 148–63. Newbury Park, CA: Sage Publications.

MacDowell, Marsha, Claire Luz, and Beth Donaldson. 2018. *Quilts and Health*. Bloomington, IN: Indiana University Press.

McIntosh, Jonathan. 2015. "Why Is the Marvel Universe—and the Geeks who Love it—Still Obsessed with Aggressive Hypermasculinity?" *Independent* November 27. https://www.independent.co.uk/voices/captain-america-civil-war-our-fixation-with-hyper-masculine-films-damages-all-of-us-a6750366.html. Last accessed May 1, 2019.

McJunkin, James N., and Max D. Crace. 1983. *Visions of Vietnam*. Novato, CA: Presidio Press.

McLay, Robert N. 2012. *At War with PTSD: Battling Post Traumatic Stress Disorder with Virtual Reality*. Baltimore, MD: The Johns Hopkins University Press.

Manning, Molly Guptill. 2015. *When Books Went to War: The Stories that Helped Us Win WWII*. Boston: Mariner Books.
March, William. 1933. *Company K*. New York: Smith and Haaas.
Markey, Patrick M., and Christopher J. Ferguson. 2017. *Moral Combat: Why the War on Violent Video Games is Wrong*. Dallas, TX: BenBella Books.
Marlantes, Karl. 2011. *What It is Like to Go to War*. New York: Atlantic Monthly Press.
Mead, Corey. 2013. *War Play: Video Games and the Future of Armed Conflict*. Boston: Houghton Mifflin Harcourt.
Mechling, Elizabeth, and Jay Mechling. 1985. "Shock Talk: From Consensual to Contractual Joking in the Workplace." *Human Organization* 44: 339–43.
———. 1988. "Play and Madness in Joseph Heller's Catch-22." *Play and Culture* 1: 226-38.
———. 1994. "The Jung and the Restless: The Mythopoetic Men's Movement." *Southern Communication Journal* 59: 97–111.
———. 1999. "American Cultural Criticism in the Pragmatic Attitude," In *At the Intersection: Cultural Studies and Rhetorical Studies*, edited by Thomas Rosteck, 137–167. New York: Guilford Press.
Mechling, Jay. 1989. "'Banana Cannon' and Other Folk Traditions between Human and Nonhuman Animals." *Western Folklore* 48: 312–323.
———. 2001. *On My Honor: Boy Scouts and the Making of American Youth*. Chicago: University of Chicago Press.
———. 2004. "Picturing Hunting." *Western Folklore* 63(1–2): 51–78.
———. 2005. "The Folklore of Mother-Raised Boys and Men." In *Manly Traditions: The Folk Roots of American Masculinities*, edited by Simon J. Bronner. 211–27. Bloomington, IN: University of Indiana Press.
———. 2008a. "The Penis." In *The Cultural History of the Body*. Vol. 2, edited by Victoria Pitts-Taylor, 384–90. Westport, CT: Greenwood Publishing.
———. 2008b. "Gun Play." *American Journal of Play* 1: 192–209.
———. 2008c. "Paddling and the Repression of the Feminine in Male Hazing." *THYMOS: Journal of Boy Studies* 2(1):60–75.
———. 2009. "Is Hazing Play?" In *Transactions at Play*, edited by Cindy Dell Clark, pp. 45–61. Lanham, MD: University Press of America.
———. 2012. "Soldier Snaps." In *Warrior Ways: Explorations in Modern Military Folklore*, edited Eric A. Eliason and Tad Tuleja, 222–47. Logan, UT: Utah State University.
———. 2014. "Pissing and Masculinity." *Culture, Society & Masculinities* 6(1): 19–34.
———. 2016. "The Erotics of Adolescent Male Altruism." *Boyhood Studies* 9(2): 92–115.
———. 2019. "Folklore and the Emotional Brain." In *Contexts of Folklore: Festschrift for Dan Ben-Amos*, edited by Simon J. Bronner and Wolfgang Mieder. New York: Peter Lang.
Messner, Michael. 1992. *Power at Play: Sports and the Problem of Masculinity*. Boston: Beacon Press.
———. 2011. *King of the Wild Suburb: A Memoir of Father, Sons, and Guns*. Austin, TX: Plain View Press.
———. 2019. *Guys Like Me: Five Wars, Five Veterans for Peace*. New Brunswick, NJ: Rutgers University Press.
Metzger, Walter P. 1963. "Generalizations about National Character: An Analytic Essay," in *Generalization in the Writing of History*, edited by Louis Gottschalk. Chicago: University of Chicago Press.
Mills, C. Wright. 1959. *The Sociological Imagination*. New York: Oxford University Press.
Mintz, Laurie. 2011. "Masturbation: Not Just Monkey Business: Masturbation is a Mentally and Physically Healthy Activity for Women." *Psychology Today* blog Jan. 31 https://www.psychologytoday.com/blog/stress-and-sex/201101/masturbation-not-just-monkey-business. Last accessed May 1, 2019.
Montalván, Luis Carlos, with Bret Witter. 2011. *Until Tuesday: A Wounded Warrior and the Golden Retriever Who Saved Him*. New York: Hyperion.

Morris, Charles E., III. 2011. *Remembering the AIDS Quilt*. Lansing, MI: Michigan State University Press.

Morris, David J. 2015a. *The Evil Hours: A Biography of Post-Traumatic Stress Disorder*. Boston: Houghton Mifflin Harcourt.

———. 2015b. "Trauma Post Trauma." *Slate* July 21.

Morris, Erroll. 2011. *Believing is Seeing: Observations on the Mysteries of Photography*. New York: Penguin Press.

Murphy, Peter F. 2001. *Studs, Tools, and the Family Jewels: Metaphors Men Live By*. Madison, WI: University of Wisconsin Press.

Myers, Jack. 2016. *The Future of Men: Masculinity on the Twenty-first Century*. Oakland, CA: Inkshares.

———. 2017. "How Media is Redefining Men and How Men are Redefining Media." *Media Village* September 5. https://www.mediavillage.com/article/how-media-is-redefining-men-and-how-men-are-redefining-media/. Last accessed May 1, 2019.

Myers, Meghann. 2018. "The Army is Tightening Waiver Authority for Recruits with Issues Like Self-mutilation, Misconduct and Substance Abuse." *Army Times* July 30. https://www.armytimes.com/news/your-army/2018/07/30/the-army-is-tightening-waiver-authority-for-recruits-with-issues-like-self-mutilation-misconduct-and-substance-abuse/. Last accessed May 11, 2019.

Nesser, John A. 2008. *The Ghosts of Thua Thien: An American Soldier's Memoir of Vietnam*. Jefferson, NE: McFarland and Company, Inc.

Obrdlik, Antonin J. 1942. "Gallows Humor"—A Sociological Phenomenon. *American Journal of Sociology* 47(5): 709–16.

O'Connell, Aaron B. 2012. *Underdogs: The Making of the Modern Marine Corps*. Cambridge, MA: Harvard University Press.

O'Donnell, M., and Sharpe, S. 2004. "The Social Construction of Youthful Masculinities: Peer Group Subcultures." In *RoutledgeFalmer Reader in Sociology of Education*, edited by S. Balla, 89–127. London: RoutledgeFalmer.

Oring, Elliott. 1984. "Dyadic Traditions." *Journal of Folklore Research* 21: 19–28.

———. 1986. "On the Concept of Folklore." In *Folk Groups and Folklore Genres*, edited by Elliott Oring, 1–22. Logan, UT: Utah State University Press.

———. 2012. "Totemism and the A.E.F. Revisited." In *Just Folklore*, 46–54. Los Angeles, CA: Cantilever Press.

Pannella, DanaMarie. 2010. "Animals are Property: The Violation of Soldiers' Rights to Strays in Iraq." *Case Western Reserve Journal of International Law* 43: 513–35.

Parnell, Sean. 2012. *Outlaw Platoon: Heroes, Infidels, and the Brotherhood of War in Afghanistan*. New York: William Morrow.

Pelligrini, Anthony. 1988. "Rough and Tumble Play and Social Competence." *Developmental Psychology*, 24: 802–06.

———. 1993. "Boys' Rough and Tumble Play and Social Competence, Contemporaneous and Longitudinal Relations." In *The Future of Play Theory*, edited by A. Pellegrini, 107–26. New York: SUNY Press.

Pieslak, Jonathan, 2009. *Sound Targets: American Soldiers and Music in the Iraq War*. Bloomington: Indiana University Press.

Pollack, Michael. 1998. *Real Boys: Rescuing Our Sons from the Myths of Boyhood*. New York: Owl Books.

Poole, Robert M. 2010. "The Pathway Home Makes Inroads in Treating PTSD." *Smithsonian Magazine* https://www.smithsonianmag.com/travel/the-pathway-home-makes-inroads-in-treating-ptsd-55062082/. Last accessed May 1, 2019.

Putney, William W. 2001. *Always Faithful: A Memoir of the Marine Dogs of WWII*. Dulles, VA: Potomac Books.

Pyszczynski, Tom, and Pelin Kesebir. 2011. "Anxiety Buffer Disruption Theory: A Terror Management Account of Posttraumatic Stress Disorder." *Anxiety, Stress, & Coping: An International Journal* 24(1): 3–26.

Ramakers, Alexis. 2017. "Timeline: A History of Service and Therapy Dogs." University of Oregon blog on Therapy and Service Dogs. https://blogs.uoregon.edu/ramakersf13gateway/timeline/. Last accessed May 1, 2019.

Raphael, Ray. 1988. *The Men from the Boys: Rites of Passage in Male America*. Lincoln: University of Nebraska Press.

Reddit. N.d. "Does Masturbation Occur in the Military? Is it non-existent?" https://www.reddit.com/r/AskReddit/comments/3ssotr/serious_does_masturbation_occur_in_the_military/ Last accessed May 1, 2019.

Remarque, Erich Maria. 1929. *All Quiet on the Western Front*. New York: Little, Brown and Company.

Reynolds, George M., and Amanda Shendruk. 2018. "Demographics of the U.S. Military." *Council on Foreign Relations* April 24. https://www.cfr.org/article/demographics-us-military. Last accessed May 1, 2019.

Rico, Johnny. 2007. *Blood Makes the Grass Grow Greener: A Year in the Desert with Team America*. San Francisco, CA: Presidio Press.

Rieckhoff, Paul. 2006. *Chasing Ghosts: A Soldier's Fight for America from Baghdad to Washington*. New York: NAL Hardcover.

Roberts, Mary Louise. 2013. *What Soldiers Do: Sex and the American GI in World War II France*. Chicago: University of Chicago Press.

Roblou, Yann. 2012. "Complex Masculinities: The Superhero in Modern American Movies." *Culture, Society & Masculinities* 4(1): 76–91.

Rockett, Ben, and Sam Carr. 2014. "Animals and Attachment Theory." *Society and Animals* 22: 415–33.

Rotunda, Kyndra Miller, and Ari Freilich. 2014. "Self-Inflicted Wounds: How Military Regulations Prejudice Service Members." *University of Massachusetts Law Review* 9(2): 424–42.

Rueckert, William H. 1982. *Kenneth Burke and the Drama of Human Relations*. Berkeley, CA: University of California Press.

Sapolsky, Robert M. 1997. *The Trouble With Testosterone and Other Essays on the Biology of the Human Predicament*. New York: Simon & Schuster.

———. 2004. *Why Zebras Don't Get Ulcers*. 3rd ed.; New York: St. Martin's Griffin.

———. 2017. *Behave: The Biology of Humans at Our Best and Worst*. New York: Penguin.

Schonauer, Scott. 2005. "Maxim Magazine to Send Free Copies to Servicemembers in Iraq." *Stars and Stripes* April 21 https://www.stripes.com/news/maxim-magazine-to-send-free-copies-to-servicemembers-in-iraq-1.32181. Last accessed May 1, 2019.

Shane, Leo, III, and Patricia Kime. 2016. "New VA Study Finds 20 Veterans Commit Suicide Each Day." *Military Times* (blog) www.militarytimes.com/story/veterans/2016/07/07/va-suicide-20-daily-research/86788332/. Last accessed May 1, 2019.

Shay, Jonathan. 1994. *Achilles in Vietnam; Combat Trauma and the Undoing of Character*. New York: Scribner.

———.2002. *Odysseus in America: Combat Trauma and the Trials of Homecoming*. New York: Scribner.

Sites, Kevin. 2013. *The Things They Cannot Say: Stories Soldiers Won't Tell You About What They've Seen, Done or Failed to Do*. New York: Harper Perennial.

Slotkin, Richard. 1973. *Regeneration Through Violence: The Mythology of the American Frontier, 1600–1860*. Middletown, CT: Wesleyan University Press.

———. 1985. *The Fatal Environment: The Myth of the Frontier in the Age of Industrialization, 1800–1890*. New York: Macmillan Publishing Co.

———. 1992. *Gunfighter Nation: The Myth of the Frontier in Twentieth-Century America*. New York: Atheneum.

Smithson, Ryan. 2009. *Ghosts of War: The True Story of a 19-Year-Old GI*. New York: HarperCollins.

Solaro, Erin. 2006. *Women in the Line of Fire*. Emeryville, CA: Seal Press.

Solomon, Sheldon, Jeff Greenberg, and Tom Pyszczynski. 2015. *The Worm at the Core: On the Role of Death in Life*. New York: Random House.

Sontag, Susan. 1966 [1965]. "The Imagination of Disaster." In *Against Interpretation and Other Essays*, 209–25. New York: Farrar, Straus and Giroux.

———. 1978. *Illness as Metaphor*. New York: Farrar, Straus and Giroux.

———. 1986. *AIDS and Its Metaphors*. New York: Farrar, Straus and Giroux.

Stearns, Carol Zisowitz, and Peter N. Stearns. 1986. *Anger: The Struggle for Emotional Control in America's History*. Chicago: University of Chicago Press.

Steinhauer, Jennifer. 2019. "V.A. Official, and the Nation, Battle an Unrelenting Tide of Veteran Suicides." April 14. https://www.nytimes.com/2019/04/14/us/politics/veterans-suicide.html. Last accessed May 1, 2019.

Steinmetz, Katy. 2017. "Beyond He or She: How a New Generation is Redefining the Meaning of Gender." *Time Magazine* March 15. http://time.com/4703309/gender-sexuality-changing/. Last accessed May 1, 2019.

Stern Stephen L., et al. 2013. "Potential Benefits of Canine Companionship for Military Veterans with Posttraumatic Stress Disorder (PTSD)." *Society and Animals* 21: 568–81.

Sullivan, Christine. 2009. *Saving Cinnamon: The Amazing True Story of a Missing Military Puppy and the Desperate Mission to Bring Her Home*. New York: St. Martin's Griffin.

Susman, Warren. 1985. *Culture as History*. New York: Pantheon.

Sutton-Smith, Brian. 1997. *The Ambiguity of Play*. Cambridge, MA: Harvard University Press.

Sutton-Smith, Brian, John Gertsmyer, and Alice Meckley. 1988. "Playfighting as Folkplay amongst Preschool Children." *Western Folklore* 47: 161–76.

Sutton-Smith, Brian, and Diana Kelly-Byrne. 1984. "The Masks of Play." In *The Masks of Play*, edited by B. Sutton-Smith and D. Kelly-Byrne, 184–99. New York: Leisure Press.

Swofford, Anthony. 2003. *Jarhead: A Marine's Chronicle of the Gulf War and Other Battles*. New York: Scribner.

Tannen, Deborah. 1990. *You Just Don't Understand: Women and Men in Conversation*. New York: William Morrow and Company.

Taylor, Myra, Julie Ann Pooley, and Mary Edwards. 2015. "Reaching Down and Finding Humanity: Military Personnel's Experiences of Adopting Dogs While on Deployment." *Society and Animals* 23: 321–42.

Theweleit, Klaus. 1989. *Male Fantasies: Vol 2, Male Bodies: Psychoanalyzing the White Terror*. Trans. Erica Carter and Chris Turner. Minneapolis, MN: University of Minnesota Press.

Thorne, Barrie. 1993. *Gender Play: Girls and Boys in School*. New Brunswick, NJ: Rutgers University Press.

Thorpe, Helen. 2014. *Soldier Girls: The Battles of Three Women at Home and at War*. New York: Scribner.

Tick, Edward. 2005. *War and the Soul: Healing Our Nation's Veterans from Post-Traumatic Stress Disorder*. Wheation, IL: Quest Books.

Tregaskis, Richard. 1955. *Guadalcanal Diary*. New York: Random House. Landmark Book #55.

Turner, Victor. 1967.*The Forest of Symbols: Aspects of Ndembu Ritual*. Ithaca, NY: Cornell University Press.

Twenge, Jean M. 2006. *Generation Me*. New York: Free Press.

———. 2017. *iGen*. New York: Atria Books.

Uriarte, Maximillian. 2016a. "Some see a shitter door. Marines see a blank canvas. Terminal Lance FaceBook page https://www.facebook.com/terminallance/photos/a.381118123607.159835.371652628607/10154550900253608/?type=3&theater. Last Accessed May 1, 2019.

———. 2016b. *The White Donkey*. New York: Little, Brown and Company.

U.S. Department of Veterans Affairs, National Center for PTSD. 2015. Dogs and PTSD. https://www.ptsd.va.gov/public/treatment/cope/dogs_and_ptsd.asp. Last accessed May 1, 2019.

———. 2019. "Traumatic Stress in Women Veterans." https://www.ptsd.va.gov/professional/treat/type/trauma_female_veterans.asp. Last accessed May 1, 2019.
van Driel, Mels. 2008. *Manhood: The Rise and Fall of the Penis*. London: Reaktion Books.
———. 2012. *With the Hand: A Cultural History of Masturbation*. Trans. Paul Vincent. London: Reaktion Books.
Van Gennep, Arnold. 1961. *The Rites of Passage*. Chicago: University of Chicago Press.
Viglianco-VanPelt, Michelle, and Kyla Boyse. 2009. "Masturbation-Your Child Developmental Behavior Resource." http://www.med.umich.edu/yourchild/topics/masturb.htm. Last accessed May 1, 2019.
Vitztum, Coley, and Julie Urbanik. 2016. "Assessing the Dog: A Theoretical Analysis of the Companion Animal's Actions in Human-Animal Interactions." *Society and Animals* 24: 172–85.
Vonnegut, Kurt. 1969. *Slaughterhouse-Five, or The Children's Crusade: A Duty-Dance with Death*. New York: Delacorte.
Wallis, John Paul. 2012. *Reborn to Kill: American Warriors and Digital Trophies*. Unpublished senior thesis in American Studies, University of California, Davis.
Wallis, John Paul, and Jay Mechling. 2015. "Devil Dogs and Dog Piles." *Western Folklore* 74: 275–308.
Ward, Jane. 2015. *Not Gay: Sex Between Straight White Men*. New York: New York University Press.
Ward, Joseph T. 1991. *Dear Mom: A Sniper's Vietnam*. New York: Ivy Books.
Warrior Canine Connection. http://warriorcanineconnection.org
Webb, James. 1978. *Fields of Fire*. New York: Prentice-Hall.
Weisbecker, A. C. 1986. *Cosmic Banditos*. New York: Vintage.
Werner, Anna. 2018. "80 Percent of Mass Shooters Showed No Interest in Video Games, Researcher Says." CBS blog March 8. https://www.cbsnews.com/news/80-percent-of-mass-shooters-showed-no-interest-in-video-games-researcher-says/ Last accessed May 1, 2019.
West, John. 2018. "Modern Masculinity." *The Marketing Insider* July 18. https://www.mediapost.com/publications/article/322314/modern-masculinity.html Last accessed May 1, 2019.
Wheeler, Evangeline A., and Margaret E. Faulkner. 2015. "The 'Pet Effect': Psychological Calming in the Presence of Canines." *Society and Animals* 23: 425–38.
Williams, Kayla, and Michael E. Staub. 2005. *Love My Rifle More than You: Young and Female in the U.S. Army*. New York: Norton.
Wolff, Tobias. 1995. *In Pharoah's Army: Memoirs of the Lost War*. New York: Vintage.
Wright, Evan. 2004. *Generation Kill: Devil Dogs, Iceman, Captain America, and the New Face of American War*. New York: Berkley.
Wright, Bradford W. 2001. *Comic Book Nation: The Transformation of Youth Culture in America*. Baltimore, MD: The Johns Hopkins Press.
Wright, Will. 1977. *Sixguns and Society: A Structural Study of the Western*. Berkeley: University of California Press.
Young, Allan. 1995. *The Harmony of Illusions: Inventing Post-Traumatic Stress Disorder*. Princeton, NJ: Princeton University Press.
Young, Matt. 2018. *Eat the Apple*. New York: Bloomsbury.
Zeeland, Steven. 1996. *The Masculine Marine: Homoeroticism in the Marine Corps*. New York: Harrington Park Press.

Index

About the Authors

John Paul Wallis was raised by a family of veterans in Hawaii. He grew up immersed in military culture. He served as an enlisted infantryman in the United States Marine Corps, with deployments to Iraq in 2007 and 2008-2009. Informed by his experiences as a Marine, he pursued understanding of conflicting perspectives about serving in a controversial war as an American studies major at UC Davis. He dedicated himself to becoming an advocate for veterans while attending UC Davis School of Law, where he worked to provide legal services to homeless veterans. He volunteered as a cofounder of a local chapter of Team RWB, a nonprofit that works to enrich the lives of America's veterans by connecting them to their community through physical and social activity. He also worked with the San Francisco Bar Association to inform Department of Defense efforts to combat military sexual assault. He currently lives in Dallas, Texas, and continues to advise his fellow veterans navigating a complex set of health, benefits, and legal issues. He and co-author Jay Mechling work together to examine folklore, memory, and masculinity among warriors in America.

Jay Mechling is professor Emeritus of American studies at the University of California, Davis. All of his degrees are interdisciplinary (BA American studies from Stetson University, MA and PhD American civilization from the University of Pennsylvania). While much of his scholarship is on masculinity and on the lives of children and youth (both topics combined in his 2001 book, *On My Honor: Boy Scouts and the Making of American Youth*, for example), he writes about a broad range of subjects and has written often with his wife, Elizabeth Walker Mechling, a rhetorical critic. He is a fellow of the American Folklore Society and has won numerous teaching awards on campus and nationally, including the Davis Prize (2006), the campus's top honor for distinguished teaching and scholarship.

Lightning Source UK Ltd.
Milton Keynes UK
UKHW021041081119
353137UK00004B/229/P

9 781793 603890